CYCLE CHARTING *for* SINGLE WOMEN

THE CATHOLIC WOMAN'S GUIDE TO CHARTING YOUR MENSTRUAL CYCLE
FOR HEALTH AND WHOLENESS

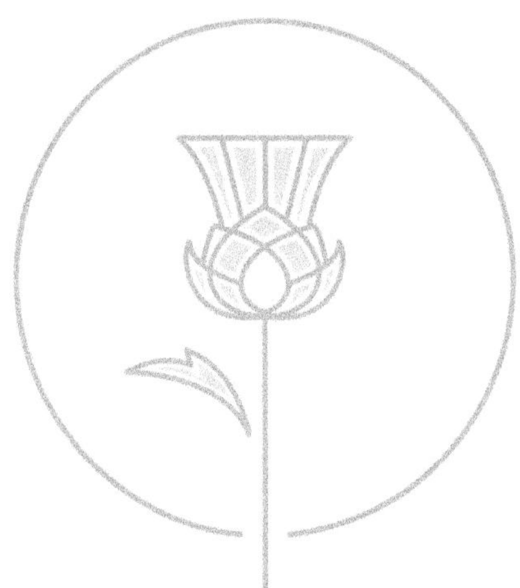

Christina Valenzuela

pearlandthistle.com

Cycle Charting for Single Women:
The Catholic Woman's Guide to Charting Your Menstrual Cycle for Health and Wholeness

Published by: Pearl and Thistle, LLC
pearlandthistle.com

ISBN: 979-8-9872139-2-6

Disclaimers: The observation techniques detailed in this guide only provide information on charting for self-knowledge. These observations are not intended to substitute for professional instruction in a fertility awareness or Natural Family Planning method. The recommendations given in this guide are not intended to replace qualified medical advice which would be particular to the individual.

This guide contains information relating to health. All efforts have been made to ensure the accuracy of the information contained in this course as of the date of publication. The author disclaims responsibility for any adverse effect arising from the use or application of the information contained herein.

Cover and Book Design by Christina Valenzuela
Pearl and Thistle, LLC

Portrait of Pope John Paul II used with permission under Creative Commons Attribution 2.0 Generic- Uploaded a work by Beyond Forgetting from https://www.flickr.com/photos/bren/8226888/. Filter applied and background removed.
Menstrual Cycle image by designua © 123RF.com, cropped and modified for font.

+AMDG+

For my family, my clients, and the many women who have shared their body literacy journeys with me as mentors, confidants, and friends

CONTENTS

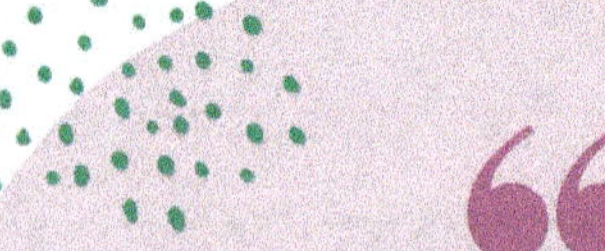

“

The human body speaks a language of which it is not the author.

- John Paul II,
Theology of the Body 104:7

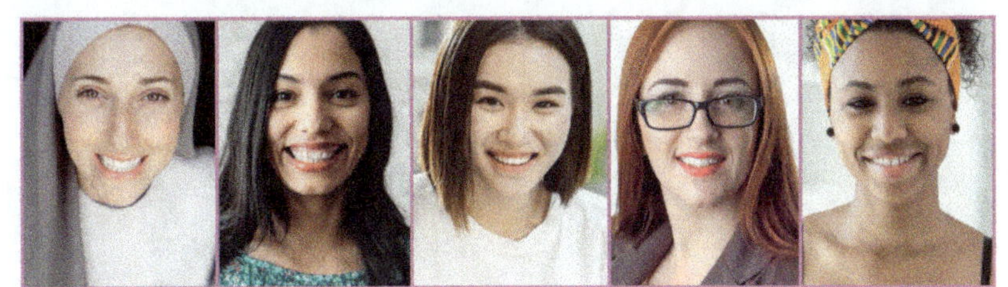

Dear Catholic Sister,

Living in a body is hard. Our bodies experience pain, sickness, and lots of discomfort. But our bodies are also the way we experience love: through physical touch, gestures, words, and in a very unique way—the Sacraments of the Church, which are God's love poured out through physical objects to give us grace. How can we awaken ourselves to the mystery of what Pope St. John Paul II called the *Language of the Body*?

I'm a Natural Family Planning (NFP)* instructor. So when I begin to ponder this question, I immediately think about where I have seen an awakening to the language of our bodies recently: cycle charting and its relationship to the term "body literacy."

For women, our cycles provide a very specific insight into the design and function of our bodies. By learning how to observe and chart our cycles, we learn to listen to the language of the female body. Rather than doing all the talking, we allow our bodies to communicate to *us* and teach us the language which we did not author. At its core, this language says:

- I am designed for communion.
- I am designed for the indwelling of life.
- I am designed to give and receive love.

When we learn to read these Truths about our female bodies, even if our periods and cycles are frustrating, it's easier for us to understand the Truth about how male and female bodies have been designed together. We see the connections between union and procreation. We see how we can use our bodies to speak the Truth, rather than speaking a lie. I believe this is particularly important because for so many women, our cycles and our feminine bodies sometimes feel like our own worst "enemies." I can't pretend that body literacy will heal the wounds some of us carry when we try to think of the goodness of our bodies, but at a minimum it will open us up to a new path of self-knowledge. And hopefully, that knowledge leads us to recognize God's image and likeness in ourselves, therefore experiencing God's love deeply in the language of our bodies.

This guide is designed to teach you the basics of charting your cycle for health, in conversation with our Catholic faith. **It will not teach you how to use all of these observations for family planning,** but will teach you the basics of cycle patterns, fertility, and how this knowledge can enhance our understanding of ourselves and our relationships: whether marriage, friendship, or the bonds of community life!

To that end, I highly encourage you to learn the habits of charting with a circle of friends. If you have the opportunity, please use this guide as part of a small group or book club, not just to strengthen your understanding of the materials, but to share in mutual discovery with others the **unique way** God has designed each of our bodies to speak His language of Love.

love, Christina

Founder of Pearl & Thistle

**the terms NFP and Fertility Awareness Based Method (FABM) are used fairly interchangeably in Catholic circles. Because I began instruction working with couples specifically for family planning, I prefer the former term, but appreciate the term FABM as well.*

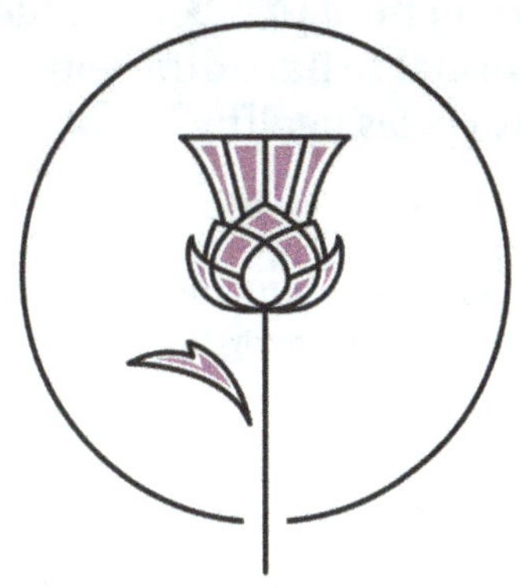

INTRODUCTION
TO CHARTING

Charting for Self-Knowledge

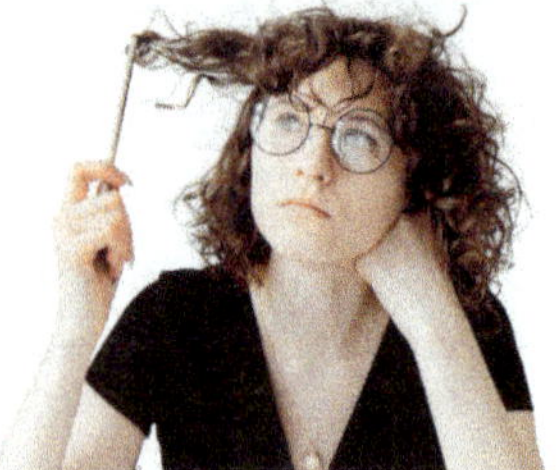

When will my next period come?
Is it possible to bleed too much? Too little?
When do I need to talk to the doctor about my cycles?
Is it normal to have different types of discharge in my underwear?
Are my cycles healthy?

As women, we tend to have lots of questions about our cycles, but most of us have been taught to either just ignore them or just accept that there aren't any real, lasting solutions.

Are your cramps awful? *Take birth control!* Your periods are too heavy? *Take birth control!* PMS is too disruptive? *Take birth control! ... When you stop taking birth control, this will probably all come back. But you don't need to worry about that until you're ready to get pregnant.*

Ladies: this is not real healthcare. Our cycles should not ONLY matter when we are trying to have a baby. To put it another way: there are not many "safe" spaces where our cycles are respected as healthy, normal, and integral to our health, despite the fact that the American College of Obstetricians and Gynecologists are calling them a "vital sign" for girls.[1]

As Catholics who believe in the goodness of our bodies, this should give us pause. This is not to say that hormonal treatments aren't necessary sometimes, but at the very least we should be seeking out the expertise of women, doctors, and specialists who can help us learn to *listen* to our bodies and respond when something seems "off," rather than trying to shove everything under the proverbial rug with birth control.

In the past, cycle charting has largely been reserved for women who want to use this knowledge for fertility and family planning. But I would like to invite all women to learn how to observe and track our cycles, so we can better learn to *read* in our body how God has designed us to function as women—like this single woman, who wrote to me a couple of years ago to share her experience of gaining body literacy to help with Irritable Bowel Syndrome (IBS):

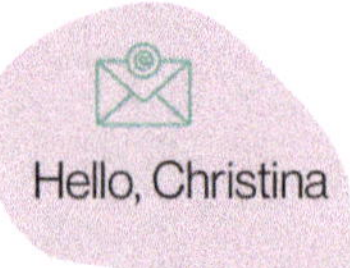

Tracking has actually been helpful with dealing with my IBS! When I first started getting sick and was asked to do a food and symptom log, I really struggled with trying to control what was happening in my body, blaming myself and blaming food, and getting very frustrated with my body. But with tracking, I feel more like I am checking in with my body and listening to what it's trying to tell me. For example, in my last cycle the confirmation for ovulation happened two days later than in previous cycles and my period subsequently came later. Our heater stopped working shortly before ovulation would have happened and I was very stressed dealing with our house being very cold, repairs, plus my normal work and life load. **I felt like I had body literacy for the first time, maybe ever. I was very stressed and my body responded and I could see the signs of that**. I am starting to work with a nutritionist because I feel I can finally apply the same mindset with tracking my IBS, which has already been helpful in dealing with symptoms. So thank you for teaching a fertility awareness method. I wish I would have learned body literacy sooner and to respect my reproductive system instead of viewing it like a hindrance and inconvenience. **It's really amazing all the female body does and I can't believe I was never taught it.**

1- American College of Obstetricians and Gynecologists: Committee on Adolescent Healthcare. Menstruation in Girls and Adolescents: Using the Menstrual Cycle as a Vital Sign, committee opinion Number 651, 2006. www.acog.org

Charting for Self-Knowledge

The implications for inviting single women to become literate about their bodies can have many potential health benefits, and I completely echo my client's sentiments that this information should be shared with us *as women who have a right to know about our bodies*—not just saved for pregnancy planning. But on an even deeper level, my mission is to also invite Catholic women to consider how becoming body literate can tell us about many aspects of life which are affected by cyclical hormones like moods, our energy levels, and even our relationships!

We'll explore some of these facets of body literacy throughout this guide, but for now I want to open with an invitation for you to think about all of those times when you've stood in front of the bathroom mirror and asked yourself: "Why am I crying right now?" or "Why am I feeling so angry?" If you're like me, these times of perceived weakness might stand out more in your memory than times of confidence, but you can also try to recall standing in front of that same mirror and saying, "I feel good today," or "Wow—my hair looks cute!"

This relates to body literacy because our hormones and cycle phases contribute to our "inner voice." In other words, hormones can play a part in shaping how we think of ourselves, especially as we relate to others—including God. I will never forget the time a friend shared with me that when she came off birth control, she finally felt like she could be *honest in her prayer life.*

> "While I was taking birth control, I felt like I never had an inner voice. Or like I was somehow restricted in what I could think or say about myself, especially when I was trying to talk to God. Once I got my natural cycle back and learned how to pay attention to that inner voice, I learned how it changed over the course of a cycle and I finally felt like I could actually express my WHOLE SELF in prayer."

Let that one sink in.

Now, let's get one thing firmly established: we are not completely controlled by our hormones, and to see our biology as something which dictates our every action would be contrary to our faith. But I like to say that we do experience different "flavors" of our personality which come out in different cycle phases, as well as varied needs in our diet, energy levels, and so much more.

So the fundamental question I pose throughout this entire guide is:

How could learning to understand and embrace cyclical changes help us become more comfortable with ourselves, as uniquely beloved daughters of God?

Charting for Self-Knowledge

If you're still reading this guide, I'm willing to bet that you're interested in learning how to chart. However, there are two important things I want to say before we dive in further:

1. While charting can be highly beneficial and even recommended in many situations, no woman is ever required to chart. It should be a choice that you make, which serves goals you have for yourself.

2. There is no one "right" way to chart. In this guide, I am offering a highly flexible set of options for you to begin with, but as you get deeper into charting, you may find that this particular methodology is not a good fit. This guide, after all, is not meant to replace formal instruction in a Natural Family Planning method, and so I expect that if you get married and want to use NFP, you will move on to something else! But you also may find that you need medical guidance, and therefore another method will be better suited for that application. You can read more about those options later on, and I highly encourage you to use this resource to begin "exploring" the world of fertility and cycle awareness. The beauty of having so many formal method options is you can find something which resonates and works FOR YOU.

KEEPING A CHART

As you begin charting, you will have many options for keeping track of your cycle. Depending on your preferences and goals, you could simply opt for tracking daily information on a calendar, or you can use one of the special charts provided in this guide. The book also contains a few app suggestions for you, if that's your preferred tracking system!

So, finally: before we get started, I'd like you to keep the following things in mind:

- It's perfectly okay not to chart—even if you have started charting, you can stop at any time. Feel free to pick up charting and put it aside whenever you want to.
- Charting for single women is all about self-knowledge and learning to appreciate your body's amazing work. If charting ever becomes something which causes you to think negatively about your body or your self, it is no longer fulfilling its purpose and it's probably in your best interest to stop charting for a while.
- There are a lot of things we can intentionally control with our bodies, but our menstrual cycle is not one of them. What we *can* control is how we respond to what our body is trying to tell us.
- Don't worry if your charts don't look exactly like the samples! Every chart is unique because every woman is unique.
- Charting may reveal some health concerns, or perhaps you already know that you have health concerns related to cycles. If you have a doctor who is willing to work with your charts, that is wonderful. If you don't, do not get discouraged! This guide contains resources to help connect you with someone who may be able to provide better health support.

Ready?? Let's begin!

Anatomy & the Menstrual Cycle

ANATOMY

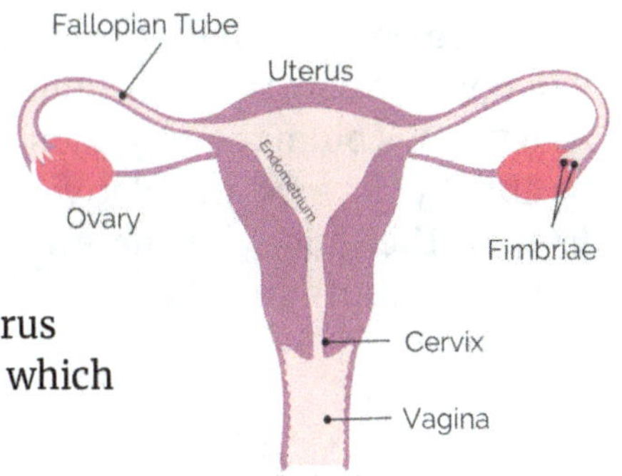

The **uterus** is a small, pear-sized organ which sits in a woman's lower abdomen. The bottom tip of the uterus is called the **cervix** (you could imagine it like the opening at the bottom of a funnel). Within the cervix, there are **crypts**—or side chambers—which produce and store **cervical fluid.** The layers of lining within the uterus are called the **endometrium.** It is the top layer of the endometrium which is built up and then shed each menstrual cycle.

The uterus has elongated tubes which protrude from either side towards the ovaries. These are the Fallopian tubes, and they are equipped with tiny finger-like projections at the end called **fimbriae.** It is within the ovaries that eggs are stored. Eggs are the female **gamete:** cells which contain half of the genetic material needed to make up a new person. Within the ovaries, eggs mature in small **follicles** (sacs). When they are released, oscillations made by the fimbriae will help the egg enter the Fallopian tube and travel towards the uterus.

THE CYCLE

It is fairly common for me to hear a woman say that she is "on her cycle" when she is experiencing a bleed; however, the words "cycle" and "period" are not synonymous. The menstrual cycle is the entire process your body goes through to prepare for the possibility of a pregnancy. Contrary to popular belief, you do not need to have a 28-day cycle in order to be considered "regular." From start to finish, a menstrual cycle can typically last from 21 to 35 days for most women and learning how to identify regularity for *your body* is a huge benefit of charting. The menstrual cycle is typically discussed in reference to four things: the events of menstruation and ovulation, and the follicular and luteal phases.

The beginning of a cycle is marked by **menstruation.** During this time, the uterus sheds the lining which had been prepared in the previous cycle. It is also called a "period" or "menses" and the bleed may last on average 3-7 days.

During the **follicular phase,** your ovary is in the process of preparing a follicle to release an egg. Estrogen gradually increases during this phase of the cycle. In conjunction with two pituitary hormones—luteinizing hormone (LH) and follicle stimulating hormone (FSH)—a spike in estrogen will signal the follicle to open and release its egg. This is called **ovulation**, and it is the key event in each cycle. No ovulation = no cycle!

After the follicle has released its egg, it remains in the ovary as a *corpus luteum*, which produces the hormone progesterone to oversee final preparations in the uterus. This is called the **luteal phase.**

CYCLE WITH OVULATION EXACTLY AT MID-POINT

Follicular phase 14 days

Luteal phase 14 days

MENSES

OVULATION

Total cycle length: 28 days

The Different Phases—First Glance

When we begin to understand the various events and phases of our cycle, a lot of new information will open up for us. In this guide, we will be learning how to chart not only our period bleeds, but also various biomarkers to identify **where ovulation is happening** in our unique cycles. This will tell us about where we are relative to the follicular and luteal phases. We will take a deeper look at this later in the guide, but here is a quick summary of some of the key differences between these different events and phases:

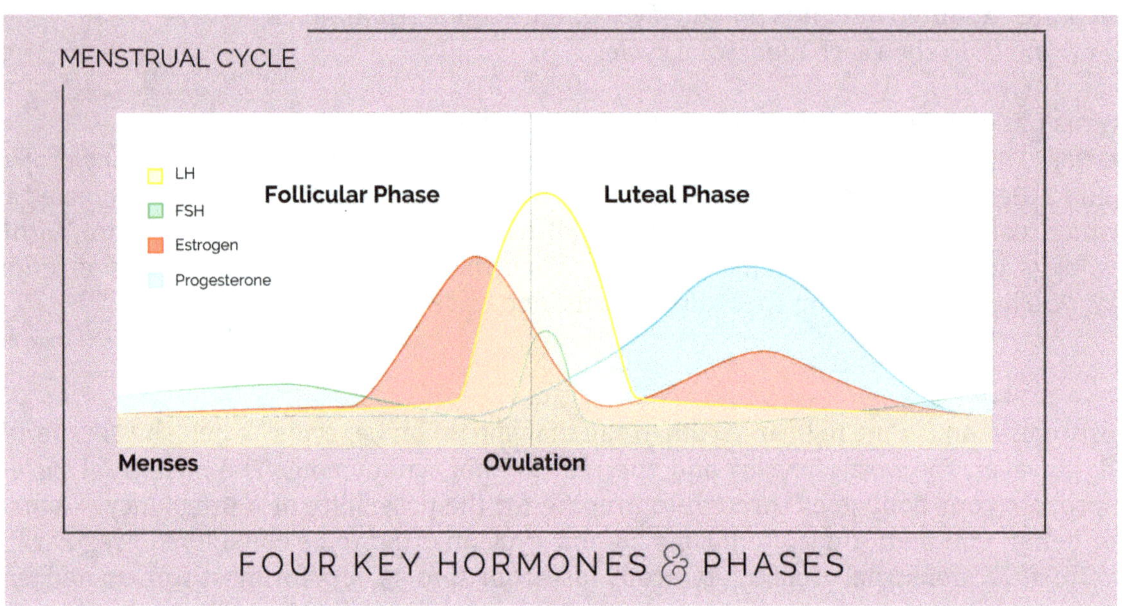

MENSTRUATION

The time when hormones are "resetting" after the last cycle. Our body spends a lot of energy expelling the top layer of endometrial lining and also preparing to begin the whole process again. The pituitary hormone, **FSH**, is already beginning to stimulate follicles within the ovaries.

FOLLICULAR PHASE

The ovarian hormone **estrogen** is working to build up a new layer of endometrial lining in the uterus. Estrogen also stimulates the cervical crypts to produce fluid. Towards the end of this phase, estrogen spikes—along with LH and FSH—to induce ovulation. Under the influence of estrogen, a woman may feel more energetic, confident, and outgoing than at other times.

OVULATION

The egg is released from its follicle. A woman may find that she experiences increased libido during the time immediately surrounding ovulation, because her body is preparing for the possibility of pregnancy. In general, this is a time when we are primed for connection with others.

LUTEAL PHASE

The follicle which released the egg now becomes the *corpus luteum* and produces **progesterone**: the pro-gestation, or pregnancy, hormone. Under the influence of progesterone, a woman's resting temperature will rise and cervical fluid production will change. In this phase, a woman may feel like her senses and emotions are heightened. She may feel inclined to rest and turn her focus slightly inward.

Understanding the "Story" of Your Cycle

If all of this still feels a little abstract to you, I'd like to introduce the idea of learning how to tell the "Story" of your menstrual cycle. This is how I teach young elementary school girls to understand all of these complicated concepts, so bear with me while I put forward a little analogy:

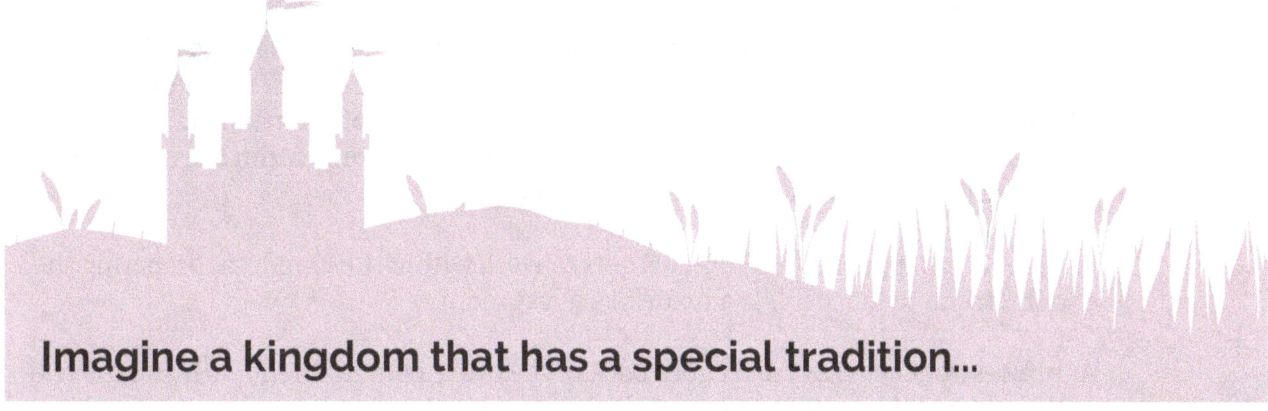

Approximately once per month, a Special Guest is invited to come and stay in the kingdom. Everyone spends time making lots of preparations, because if the Guest decides to stay, it will become the new Prince or Princess of the kingdom!

THE CAST OF CHARACTERS

FSH (Follicle-Stimulating Hormone) is like the "messenger" which invites the guest to wake up and get ready to come to the kingdom!

ESTROGEN is like the "royal steward" who oversees the beginnings of the cycle process. It produces cervical fluid and begins to thicken the endometrial lining.

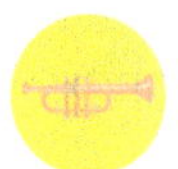

LH (Luteinizing Hormone) is like the "herald," which pairs with its friend FSH to tell the egg to exit the follicle and begin its journey in the Fallopian tube!

PROGESTERONE is like the "queen" hormone, who oversees the final preparations and takes command of work at the end of the cycle. Under her influence, body temperature is slightly elevated, cervical fluid will change and dry up, and the endometrial lining continues to change to prepare for the guest.

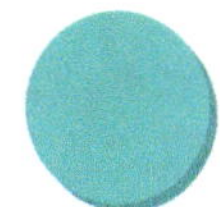

The EGG (Ovum) is the "main character" in our menstrual cycle story! The egg cell is going to play the role of "Special Invited Guest." If it does not meet with a sperm cell, the egg cell is no longer viable after 12-24 hours.

Understanding the "Story" of Your Cycle

THE STORY

Each cycle begins with a **MENSES** (period bleed).

Dear egg, wake up!

A few days into this new cycle, the messenger **FSH** visits the ovaries and delivers a special invitation from the kingdom: *One of you eggs will be invited to come and stay! It's time to wake up and start getting ready!* Eventually, one of them will be selected to mature within a follicle, which is like a special dressing room within the ovary. The egg prepares to go on its journey to the kingdom.

While this is happening, **ESTROGEN** gets to work within the kingdom, preparing the endometrium to make it like a luxurious guest room.

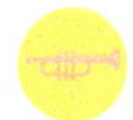

At peak estrogen activity, FSH goes back to the ovary with its friend, **LH**, and the two of them signal the egg to leave the follicle and go to the kingdom!

When the follicle opens, this is called **OVULATION.**

The follicle will then turn into the yellow *corpus luteum* and signal **PROGESTERONE** to come on the scene! Back in the uterus, progesterone will see to her queenly duties of making final preparations in the guest room. She will wait patiently for the Special Guest to arrive.

If the equation of life has taken place (the egg has met up with a sperm cell), then a baby will travel down the Fallopian tube and take up residence within the special guest room. However, in the vast majority of cases, the equation of life will NOT have happened, and the egg will dissolve before it ever reaches the kingdom.

Progesterone will wait for about 10-16 days to see if the Special Guest is coming. After that amount of time, she will tell everyone to clean up and clear out so they can begin preparing for the next guest! A new cycle begins, and repeats....

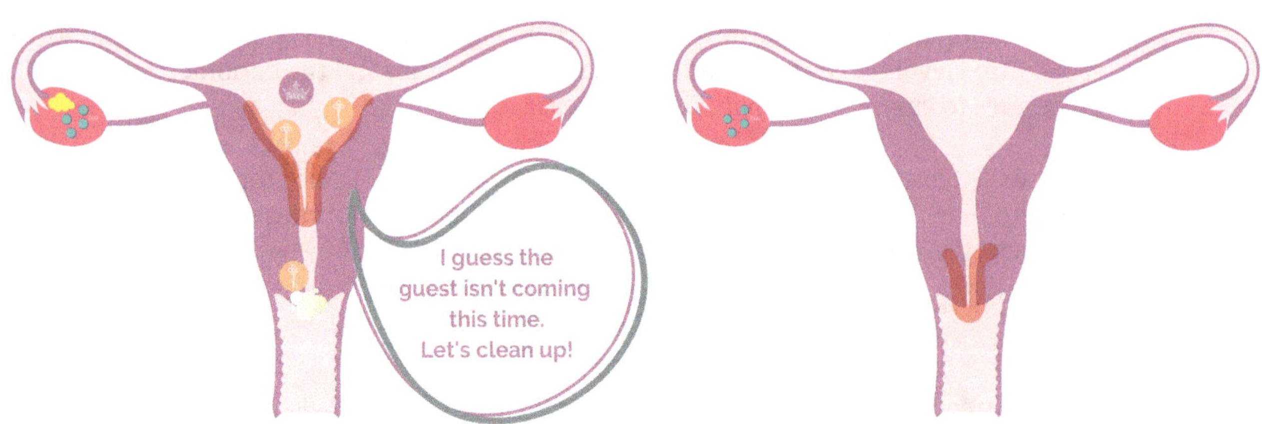

Receiving the Gift of Self-Knowledge

Before we close this section, it's worth mentioning that for many of us, learning to embrace the "goodness" of our bodies is itself a steep learning curve. For as long as we can remember, society has been showing us images of hyper-sexualized, fantasy women—telling us both implicitly and sometimes explicitly that our worth is based on how well we live up to their standard of beauty.

To combat this hyper-sexualized image, our Church has often veered in the other direction: focusing on how the body contributes to lust, impurity, and many temptations to sin. We hear St. Paul preach about the weakness or sinfulness of *the flesh,* and are often taught to equate it with our physical being. Admittedly, this sort of interpretation would make it almost impossible for us to engage positively with our bodies in the way I am suggesting. How can our faith claim that our fleshy bodies are "good"?

This particular guide is not going to offer a detailed theological treatise on the figurative meaning of "the flesh" in Biblical literature. If you are interested in a deep dive, I will highly recommend taking a romp through JPII's *Theology of the Body,* audiences 50-57, just for a start. But since you're reading here and deserve at least a quick answer, I'd like to offer a couple of quotes for you to take to prayer if you find yourself struggling to find where body positivity and body literacy can fit reverently into our Catholic faith.

In *Gaudium et spes*, one of the four constitution documents which were written as a result of the Second Vatican Council, we read:

> A person, made in the image and likeness of God, is both body and soul. For this reason, men and women are not allowed to despise bodily life, rather we are obliged to regard our bodies as good and honorable since God has created them and will raise our bodies up on the last day. The very dignity of humankind postulates that we are called to glorify God in our bodies.
> –cf. *Gaudium et spes* § 14—text amended to be gender inclusive

Perhaps not surprisingly, JPII echoes the centrality of our bodies in God's design, specifically as a means God has derived for us to receive Creation, ourselves, and God as a gift:

> In some way, therefore—even if in the most general way—the body enters into the definition of a sacrament, which is "a visible sign of an invisible reality." ... In this sign—and through this sign—God gives himself to man in his transcendent truth and in his love.
> –*TOB* 87:5

In other words, if our Catholic faith did not uphold the goodness and dignity of the body, we would have nothing positive to say about human nature, the Incarnation, or the Sacraments. Sisters, God has created you—your WHOLE self—as a gift. And He invites you to receive Himself—His WHOLE self: body, blood, soul, and divinity—through that same body. It's perfectly alright to take your time absorbing that fact. But I pray that you will be able to receive the gift of your self, because it was lovingly given by your Father, and deserves to be cherished.

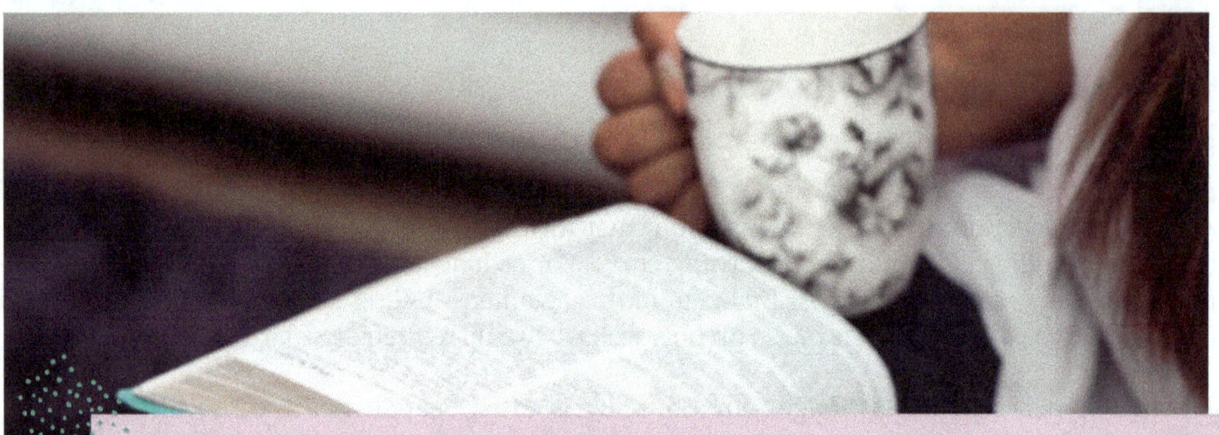

Reflection/Discussion Questions

Before we proceed to learning about how to chart and interpret our cycles, let us take time to reflect on the design of our bodies.

- Have I learned anything new about my cycles? If so, how does that make me feel?
- Is it easy for me to see that my cycles and periods are "good"? It is easy for me to see that my body, itself, is good? If so, how do I think charting can lead me to deeper appreciation of these things? If not, what are the concerns or obstacles that make it hard to see this aspect of my body as good?
- Reflect on the quotes below. Which one speaks to you as you think about your cycles & periods through this lens of the *language of the body*?

"This is the true purpose of anatomy: to lead the audience by the wonderful artwork of the human body to the dignity of the soul and by the admirable structure of both to the knowledge and love of God."
–Bl. Nicholas Steno (17th c. bishop and scientist)

"God created mankind in His image; in the image of God He created them, male and female He created them.... God looked at everything He had made, and found it very good. Evening came, and morning followed —the sixth day."
–Genesis 1:27, 31

"You formed my inmost being;
you knit me in my mother's womb.
I praise you, because I am
wonderfully made;
wonderful are your works!
My very self you know.
My bones are not hidden from you,
When I was being made in secret,
fashioned in the depths of the earth.
Your eyes saw me unformed;
in your book all are written down;
my days were shaped, before one
came to be."

–Psalm 139: 13-16

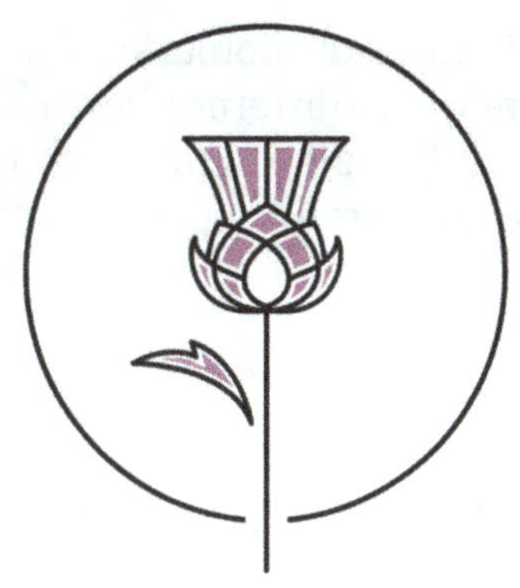

HOW TO
KEEP A CHART

Charting Cycle Biomarkers

Now that we understand the process of the cycle itself, let's talk about the things we can observe in our bodies which tell us what part of the cycle we are in. These are called *cycle biomarkers.*

In this guide, we will learn a combination of biomarkers to help us identify ovulation and the phases of the cycle. Because there are many different hormones at play which act in the body to produce different effects, there are many options for biomarkers to track. The biomarkers you choose to utilize long-term for cycle charting will depend on a few things. Some considerations will be:

1. Your personal preferences
2. Your lifestyle
3. Your information goals
4. The amount of time you want to spend each day or each cycle tracking cues
5. Your financial situation
6. Whether certain biomarkers are supported by your method (for NFP or diagnostic work)

I want to reiterate that we are not learning a full NFP method in this guide. What we will learn are observations based on the method that I teach, but modified for simplicity and utility for single women. Learning to observe, chart, interpret, and apply protocols for family planning requires a level of personal support that cannot be offered in a book.

Even though we are not learning a full method, it is still important to understand *why* and *how* specific biomarkers can be used either alone or in combination to put together a "picture" of your cycle. Let's look at the biomarker options that are typically used by NFP methods. The color blocks on the charts below indicate which part of the cycle you are able to track with each of the following biomarkers, based on the specific hormone activity they reflect:

Cervical Fluid

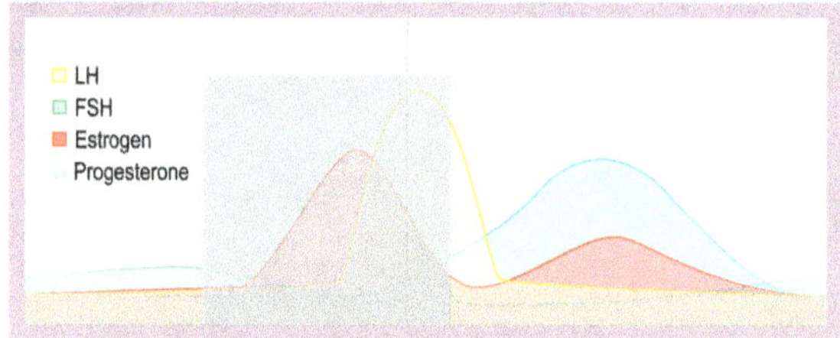

primarily tracks estrogen activity, leading up to ovulation

Temperature (BBT)

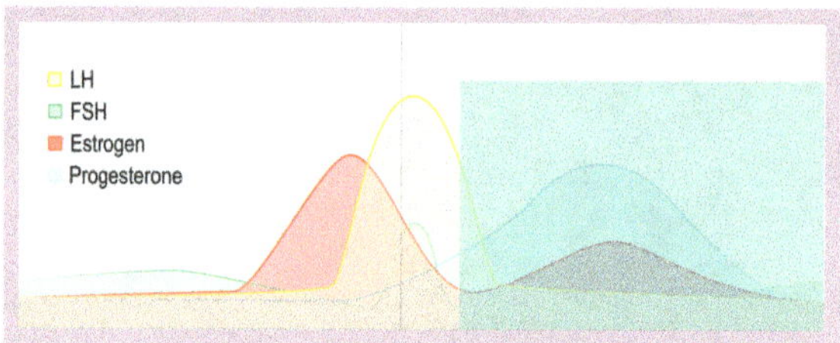

tracks progesterone activity, confirming ovulation

Additional options commonly used are hormone monitors to track estrogen + LH, or PdG tests which track the presence of progesterone

LH Tests (Ovulation Predictor Kits)

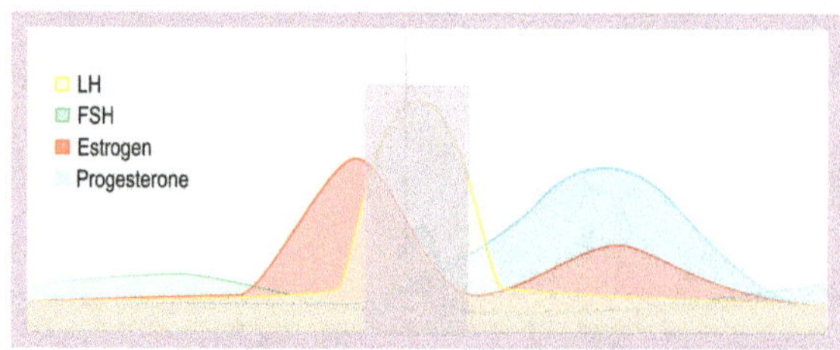

track luteinizing hormone, leading up to ovulation

Charting Cycle Biomarkers

There are many different ways to combine biomarkers, and many different reasons why you might want to choose some over others. As shown on the previous page, you could opt to simply work with one biomarker as you get started. But let's take a quick look at how the different biomarkers in this guide can be combined:

Fluid + Temps + LH

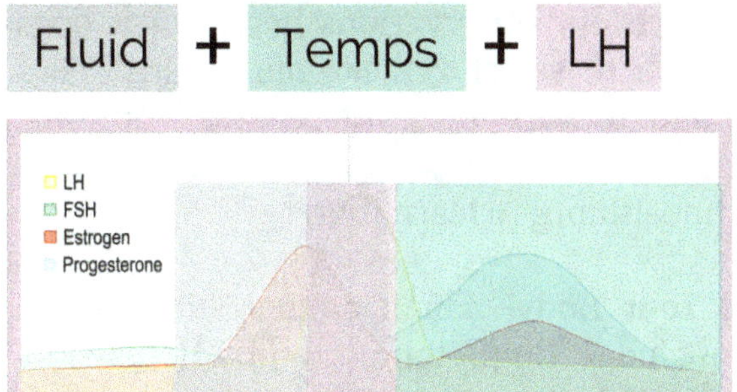

Using all three of the biomarkers in this guide will build a really robust picture of what's going on in your whole cycle. By tracking three different hormones, you get to see the relationships between them all: How quickly does estrogen production lead to an LH surge? How quickly do my temperatures respond to that surge?

Temps + LH

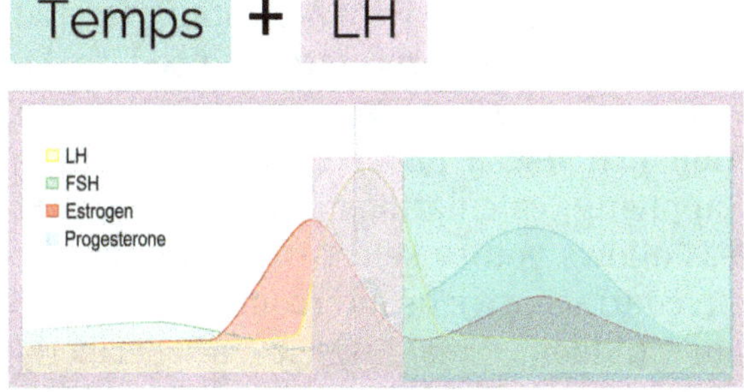

This is not a combination that would typically be used for family planning, because it does not include any estrogenic biomarkers which give advance information about upcoming ovulation, but it is a great combination for women who just want a good look at where ovulation is happening and to confirm that it has occurred.

Fluid + Temps

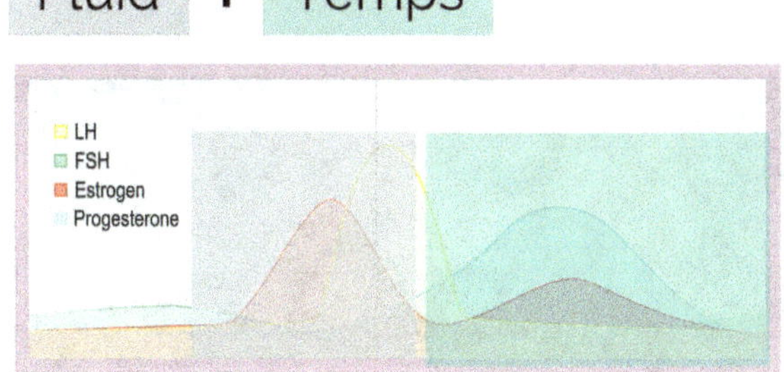

This is a classic "sympto-thermal" approach: the *sympto* comes from the fluid sign, and the *thermal* comes from the temperature sign. This is a great combination to get the simplest view of one hormone leading up to ovulation (estrogen) and one hormone confirming ovulation (progesterone).

Fluid + LH

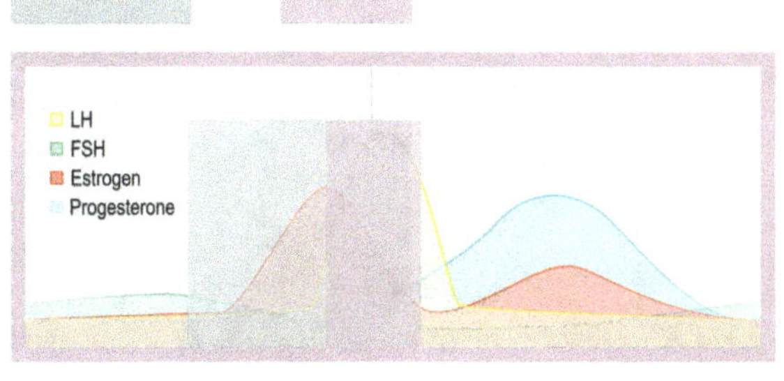

Though fluid + LH doesn't include a sign which confirms ovulation (i.e., temperature), it can still be a very good system because looking at two biomarkers can provide a high degree of confidence that ovulation is occurring in any given cycle.

Keeping a Chart in an App

There are many different ways to keep a cycle chart, and the landscape of app options seems to change daily. It may be tempting to just pick up an app and keep a chart with whatever free software you can find, but I would like to caution about a few things:

01. Charting is not standardized: terms may be different in apps from what we learn here, and not all apps will include the specific biomarkers that you want to track.

02. Most apps have predictive and/or interpretive features. Learning how to understand and interpret your own cycle data is an important step when you're looking to grow in body literacy. While this may not be as crucial for single women who aren't using this data for family planning, ensuring charting autonomy now can make a big difference long-term, because NFP requires users to learn how to do fertility calculations ***per the protocols of their method.*** I highly recommend having an app that allows you to mark interpretations for yourself.

03. Many apps have limited data privacy, so just be sure you are familiar and comfortable with all privacy policies.

04. Many apps have additional features that can make the user experience uncomfortable for single, Catholic women to chart. These can include artificial insemination, emergency contraceptives, condoms, or other options which are not compatible with the Church's teachings on sex and marriage. It is important to choose a charting system that respects your views and feels comfortable for you to spend time on each day.

That being said, there are two apps which I will frequently recommend:

FEMMHealth- free, includes fluid, temps, and LH tests by default. The fluid categories will not match our observations here, but it does allow you to select "track your health" as a goal and to turn off "intercourse" options, which are both nice features. Visit femmhealth.org to learn more!

Read Your Body- small annual subscription fee, includes fluid, temps, and LH tests by default. This is my favorite app because it guarantees total data privacy and is completely customizable, meaning you can set up your chart to work perfectly with our categories and options here. All interpretations need to be done manually by the user, making the app function just like a paper chart for learning and applying calculations. The onboarding process allows you to select if you would like certain contraceptive or intercourse options to remain hidden, making it a perfectly comfortable platform to navigate. Visit readyourbody.info to learn more!

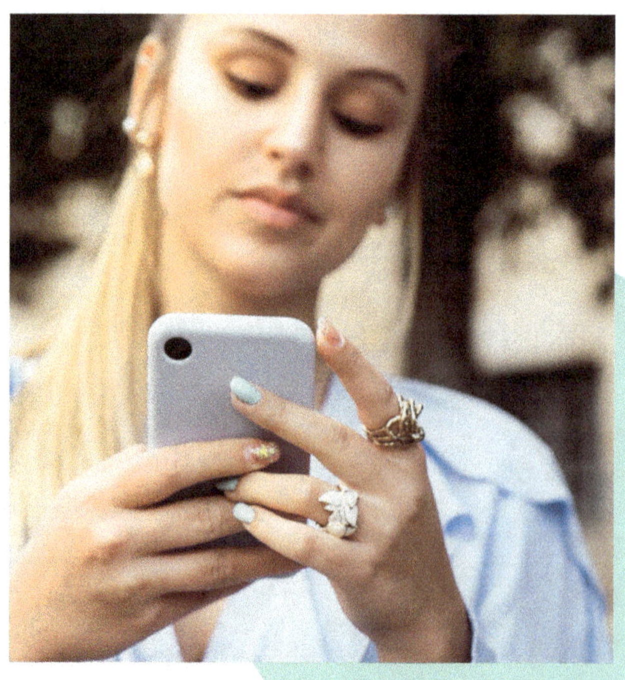

Keeping a Paper Chart

If you prefer to keep a paper chart, look no further! This is the full chart that we will use for our system. In addition to tracking bleeding day, **the three key ovulation indicators we will learn how to chart are FLUID, TEMPERATURES, and LH TESTS.** A blank version of this full chart is located at the end of this guide, so you can easily make copies whenever you need them. You will also find a chart with the temperature section removed, in case you only want to track LH and/or fluid.

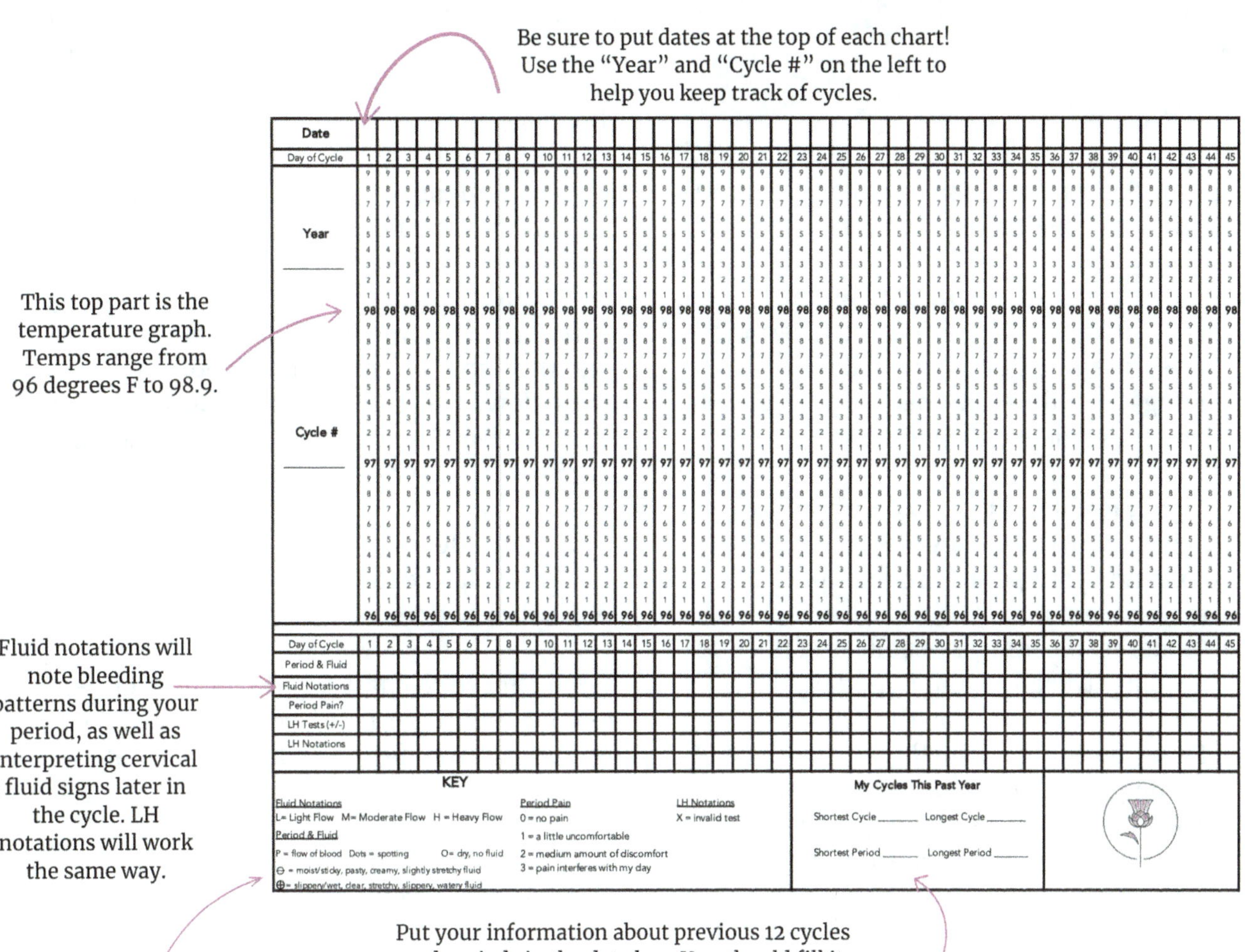

This key gives you all the notations we'll use. We'll explain about each of these features in the following pages.

Pro Tip: when you first start charting, use pencil so you can easily adjust observations as you learn!

BLEEDING DAYS: Recording on a Chart

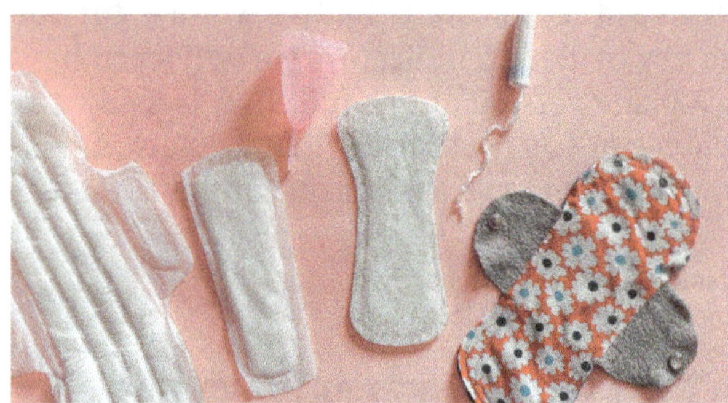

Your period (or menses, or menstruation) will mark the beginning of your new cycle.

A period starts with a **flow of blood** which can be light, moderate, or heavy. These terms are relative, meaning that they can have different meanings for different people. If you are looking for guidelines, you could say:

- **Light bleeding** is usually described as being able to go 6+ hours without changing your period product (pad, tampon, etc.).
- **Moderate bleeding** is usually described as needing to change your period products every 4-6 hours during the day.
- **Heavy bleeding** is usually described as needing to change your period products every 2 hours during the day, or needing to get up in the middle of the night.

Spotting is a different sort of bleeding, which means that you may see drops of blood when you wipe, or see a dappled red effect in your underwear. To a certain extent, learning how to identify spotting versus flow is not very important unless you are working with a practitioner for cycle issues. So don't feel like you need to obsess about this, but if wearing a panty liner is sufficient to contain the blood, then it's likely spotting rather than flow.

Spotting does not count as "flow" when we are charting our periods. So if you see spotting, it does not yet count as the start of a new cycle.

Every bleed should be recorded on your chart. Working with the paper chart, you will record all of your flow days with a "P." If you have spotting, you can put dots in the box. Note that spotting may happen before the start of a period, at the tail end of a period, or sometimes in the middle of a cycle. Regardless of when it happens, all bleeding should be marked.

It is recommended that you also keep track of how heavy your flow was each day. A typical period bleed will follow a simple crescendo-decrescendo pattern, meaning that it may start out light or moderate, progress to heavy, and then taper off after that. If you choose to mark flow, use the "Fluid Notation" boxes right under the line marked "Period and Fluid." You can write:

- L = light flow
- M = moderate flow
- H = heavy flow

If you choose to chart any discomfort or pain you feel with periods, you can put those numbers in the next line down. The scale we use is:

- 0 = no pain
- 1 = a little uncomfortable
- 2 = moderate discomfort
- 3 = pain interferes with my day

Note:
For adult women, periods typically last from 3-7 days (5 is average). Over the course of a period, a woman will typically lose about 2-4 tablespoons of blood (about 30-60 mL). If you are concerned about the amount of bleeding you experience, you can use a graduated menstrual cup or keep track of the number + type of products you use over the course of a period to estimate volume.

CERVICAL FLUID: What is it?

As we go throughout our cycle, the hormone estrogen will help the body produce different types of **cervical fluid.** Cervical fluid is also often called cervical mucus, but as an instructor I find that particular word to be off-putting, so I will refer to "fluid" throughout. Just keep in mind that it is a form of healthy mucus, and the terms refer to the same thing.

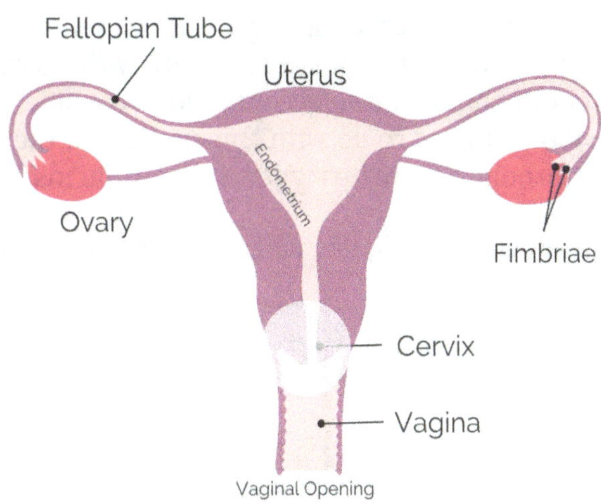

You may have already guessed from the name, but cervical fluid is a type of normal vaginal discharge which is made within the **cervix.** Among its many other functions, cervical fluid helps keep your body free from infection. It is a sign that your body is healthy. But the cervical fluid doesn't just stay up in the cervix: it will make its way out the opening and down into the vagina, where it will eventually come out of the vaginal opening. You may notice a lot of fluid or a little bit of fluid when you go to the bathroom, or as a sensation throughout the day.

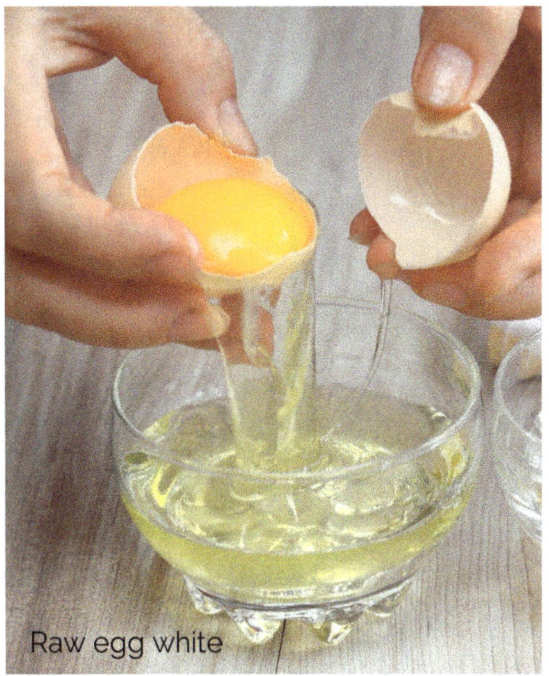

Cervical fluid is the biomarker which has the highest variations in terminology, observation techniques, and interpretation amongst different methods of NFP. We will learn a very basic categorization schema for fluid in this guide, but some methods are much more detailed, while others may be just as simple as what you learn here, just categorized differently.

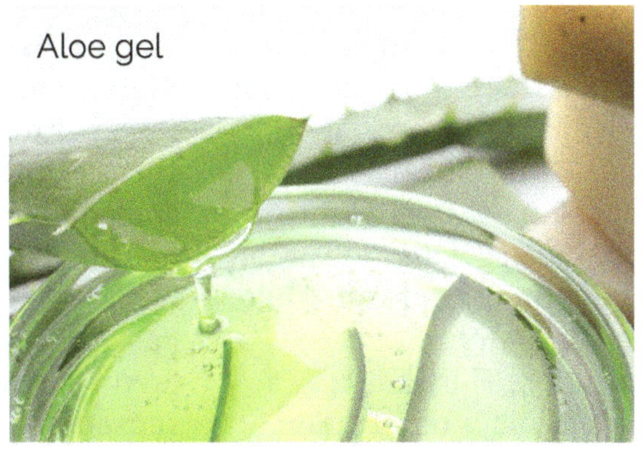

Generally all NFP methods will be looking to identify approaching ovulation by watching for the appearance of a type of cervical fluid that looks a lot like a raw egg white: it is clear, and has a stretchy, wet, slippery texture. Every woman is different, though, so you may find that your fluid is more watery. Some people also compare it to aloe gel, or simply as a feeling of being "wet."

Just remember: cervical fluid is a good sign of the work your body is doing. It is normal to see changes in this fluid throughout your cycle—and in fact, it's a very powerful and helpful sign to identify ovulation!

CERVICAL FLUID: Making Observations

Before going to the bathroom, you will use either clean fingertips or toilet paper to gently wipe front-to-back across the surface around the vaginal opening. For some women, it can be difficult to begin to observe this sign, either because it's hard to remember to check before you urinate or because there is some discomfort with observing your vulvar area. Your personal comfort level should be taken into account when considering whether to use this sign, but just remember: the wipe you need to do with this method is the same as if you were wiping after having gone to the bathroom. You're just wiping away fluid instead of urine, both of which are normal and healthy.

When you do this, you will ask yourself two questions: What do I feel? and What do I see?

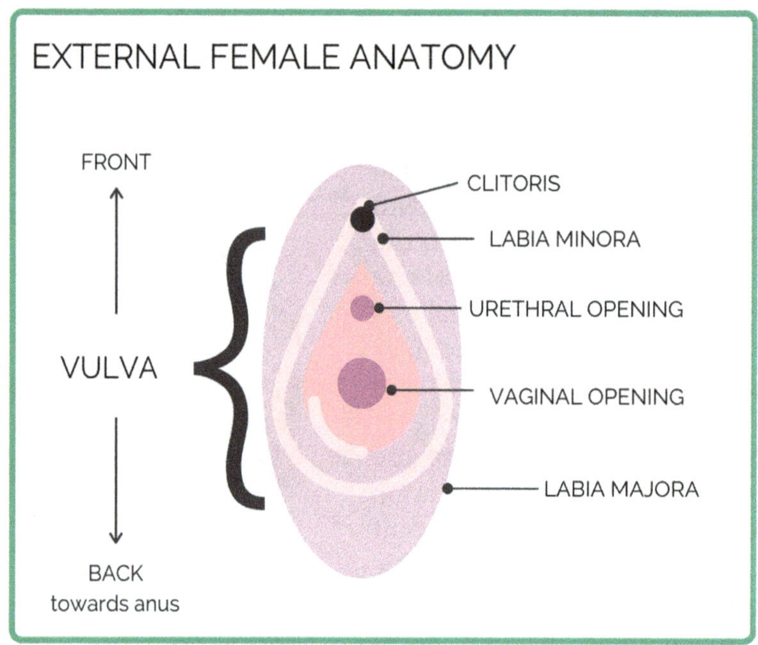

What Do I Feel? = Touch Sensation

What does it feel like when you take your fingertip or toilet paper over the vaginal opening? We will have **three different key words** for this sensation:

DRY

It doesn't feel like anything extra is there. If you are using toilet paper to check, it may drag a little bit. Sometimes your skin may feel a little dry (like if you get dry skin in the winter time!) and that would also be a "dry" sort of sensation. This should be a fairly obvious observation.

MOIST

You feel like there is something there. When you move your finger or toilet paper over the surface, it feels like you may be spreading a smooth substance like hand lotion, or it may feel like there is something tacky or pasty on your skin. If you aren't sure what sort of sensation you're feeling, it's often a "moist" category!

WET

There is something there, and it feels like a Slip 'n Slide! Your finger or toilet paper will glide easily over the surface and it will feel watery or wet. This should be a very obvious observation. Some women even feel "wet" just during the day, to the extent that they need to wear a pantyliner.

CERVICAL FLUID: Making Observations

What Do I See? = Take a look!

Then, look at your fingertips or toilet paper. What do you see? You can observe a lot of different things about your cervical fluid:

COLOR

- yellow
- white
- cloudy (like wax paper)
- clear

TEXTURE
What is it like?

- pasty= like toothpaste or a glue stick
- creamy= like smooth hand lotion
- slippery= like aloe, or a raw egg white

STRETCH
If you hold it in your fingers, does it stretch at all?

- tacky= no stretch at all
- slightly stretchy= it stretches, but only about 1/4 of an inch
- stretchy= stretches more than 1/4 of an inch

Having trouble figuring out cervical fluid categories? Visit **cervicalmucus.org** to see some examples!

GIVE EACH OBSERVATION A CATEGORY

Each time you make an observation, you'll want to ask yourself what sort of category the fluid would fall in to. Each category has particular key words taken from the lists above. Here are the key words associated with each category:

CATEGORY	WHAT I FEEL	WHAT I SEE
○ DRY	Dry	Nothing
⊖ NON-PEAK	Moist, damp, sticky, smooth	Yellow, white, cloudy, pasty, creamy, tacky, slightly-stretchy
⊕ PEAK TYPE	Wet, slippery, watery	Clear, slippery, stretchy

What if I get two different categories?

Sometimes, you will have fluid that doesn't fit very neatly into these categories. You may have something that looks cloudy, but is pretty stretchy. "Cloudy" is a key word for the Non-Peak [⊖] category, but "stretchy" is a key word for the Peak Type [⊕] category. When this happens, it's ok! Default to the category that is **lower** on the chart, because that indicates higher potential fertility. So if the options are Dry or Non-Peak, you choose Non-Peak. If the options are Non-Peak or Peak Type, you choose Peak Type.

CERVICAL FLUID: Recording on a Chart

Gather your feeling and sight observations throughout the day. Ideally, you'd check every time you use the bathroom; but if that's not feasible, then be sure to check first thing in the morning, right before bed, and maybe one or two other times. At the end of the day, you'll choose how to categorize the whole day ... and you'll categorize by the **designation that is lowest on the chart,** regardless of when that happened throughout the day.

So, if you had three observations throughout the day that were: Non-Peak, Peak Type, Non-Peak—you'd categorize that day as "Peak Type" because that category is lower on the chart. If you have four observations which are: Non-Peak, Dry, Dry, Dry—that day is "Non-Peak"

Let's do some practice:

EXTRA NOTES:

1) Looking in your underwear will not tell you about the type of fluid that you are having, because all fluid will change consistency and dry out when exposed to air. So you have to do the check on the surface of the skin.

2) Using panty liners, scented toilet paper, or period panties will impact your observations. If you need to use a panty liner because you feel wet, that is a **Peak Type** day! If you need to wear period panties because you are on your period, there is no need to check your fluid.

3) Sometimes when we experience heightened sexual arousal, we produce a type of fluid which is lubricative and can mimic the "wet" sensation. This is made by a different hormone, oxytocin. Do not count sensation observations within 60 minutes of noticeable arousal.

For each example, identify the category for each individual observation, and then identify the category for the whole day.

Check your answers at the end of this book.

Tuesday

	Observation Category:
6:30 AM- moist, pasty white fluid	______________
12 noon- moist, creamy white fluid	______________
4:00 PM- wet, creamy white fluid	______________
9:00 PM- wet, stretchy clear fluid	______________

Today's category is: ___________

Wednesday

	Observation Category:
7:00 AM- wet, stretchy clear fluid	______________
11:00 AM- wet, no fluid	______________
3:30 PM- wet, no fluid	______________
9:00 PM- wet, stretchy clear fluid	______________

Today's category is: ___________

Thursday

	Observation Category:
6:30 AM- moist, creamy white fluid	______________
11:00 AM- moist, no fluid	______________
3:30 PM- dry, no fluid	______________
9:00 PM- dry, no fluid	______________

Today's category is: ___________

BASAL BODY TEMPS: Options for Observing

Basal Body Temperature (BBT) is the measurement of your temperature when you are fully at rest. During the follicular phase, your BBT is relatively low. During the luteal phase, your BBT is a little bit higher due to the presence of progesterone. If you are consistent about taking your temperature, you can verify that ovulation has happened simply by recording this slight shift in your resting temperature.

Traditionally, BBT has been observed either orally or vaginally. Modern options for BBT thermometers range from simple inexpensive devices to fancy Bluetooth-compatible devices with associated apps. There is no need to spend lots of money: the simpler devices can be very accurate. Just be sure the thermometer you get is labeled as a "BBT Thermometer," because:

1. They are very accurate. A proper basal body thermometer will give you temperature readings accurate to the hundredths of a degree (two decimal points)
2. They often come with a memory recall feature to show you what the last temperature was. This means you can take your temperature without having to chart it right away.

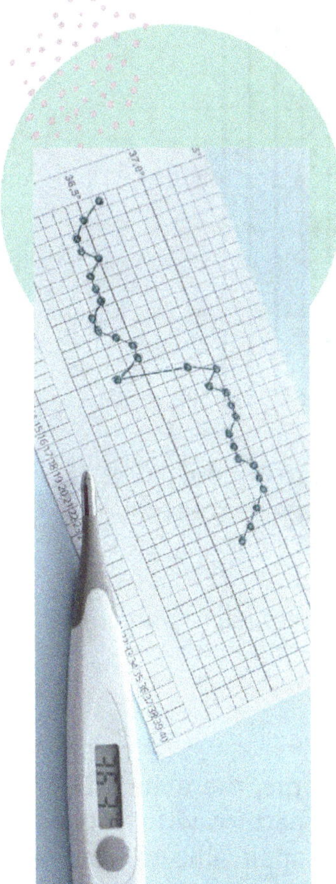

ORAL/VAGINAL BBT OBSERVATION

Keep your thermometer near your bed, because you'll need to take your temperature right when you wake up—before you get up or do anything that might affect your temperature (like drink a glass of water). It is important that you have had at least 3-4 hours of good, uninterrupted sleep prior to taking your temperature in order to ensure that your body has rested enough to get an accurate measurement.

Take your temperature at the SAME TIME each day to be the most accurate. This is called your **Base Time.** Try to get your Base Time accurately at least five days each week. If you don't manage to get your temperature at your Base Time, you can do one of two things:

1. Chart the temperature anyway. Make note of the different time somewhere on your chart so you know why that temperature may be higher or lower compared to the others around it.
2. Record an adjusted temperature. We'll learn how to make adjustments later in this guide.

NEW DEVICE OPTIONS

Traditional research for temperature calculations is based on getting oral or vaginal BBT readings; however, the advent of wearable health-monitoring devices is opening up new options for temperature observation. Official methods of NFP will often have limits about which devices are approved for protocol use, so be aware that investing in a fancy device is not always going to be the preferred option for family planning. But if you want (or need) to forego the timing restrictions which are inherent in using traditional BBT, you could opt for a wearable device which is able to give you an overnight temperature. *Please see the resource page at the back of this guide for details on a few of these devices.*

BASAL BODY TEMPS: Recording on a Chart

Even though your thermometer is accurate to two decimal points, we will only chart to one decimal point (to the tenths). The easiest way to do this is to just cut off the last number, which is referred to as *truncation:*

- If your thermometer reads 97.83°, then put a dot at 97.8 on the chart.
- If your thermometer reads 97.88°, then put a dot at 97.8 on the chart.

Each day, connect your new dot to the day before it, and you'll make a nice graph!

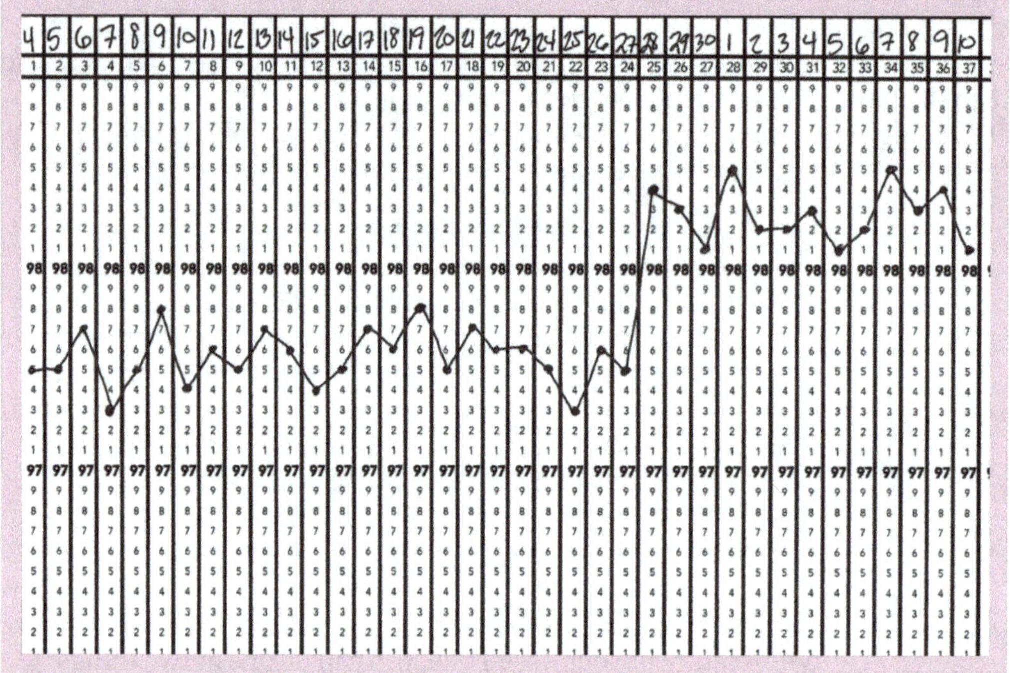

You could also use scientific rounding if you prefer that approach. The key is just to be consistent. If you are charting with an app, be sure that you are marking temps to the tenth of a degree and you know whether those temperatures are truncated or rounded.

Note: Thermometers can be calibrated differently, so it is best not to switch thermometers until the beginning of a new cycle!

WHAT MIGHT DISTURB MY TEMPERATURES?

Even though we try our best to get consistent sleep and wake up at the right time, there are still things which may throw off our temperature readings. If you notice an odd pattern with your temperatures, think about these possible culprits, and make note of them where applicable on your chart:

- Stress, which can disrupt sleep
- Fever (it is best to not temp when you know you are sick with fever)
- Alcohol consumption, which can elevate temperatures
- Use of a heating pad or blanket overnight
- Drastically different sleeping environment temperatures

BASAL BODY TEMPS: Recording on a Chart

ADJUSTING TEMPERATURES

If you are unable to get your temperature at your base time, you can adjust temperatures using the techniques below. If you do this, always note on your chart what time you woke up and what your original temperature reading was. If you are using paper charts, notes can easily be written on the back of the sheet. If you are using an app, a note or journal feature is fairly standard. Chart the adjusted temperature on the graph. This is not a perfect solution and does not always yield clear results, but it is better than recording temperatures which we know were not taken at the base time.

WHY DOES THIS WORK?

After hitting your lowest temperature of the night, your body raises its temperature by about a tenth of a degree (one decimal point) every HALF HOUR as your body prepares to wake up. So we can approximate what your temperature would have been by adjusting the data a tenth of a degree for every half hour of difference between your wake up time and your base time.

For every half hour you sleep in, you will therefore need to subtract 0.1 to get back to what your temp **would have been** at your Base Time. For every half hour you get up early, you add 0.1 **to predict** what your temp would have been at your Base Time. Use the chart below to help!

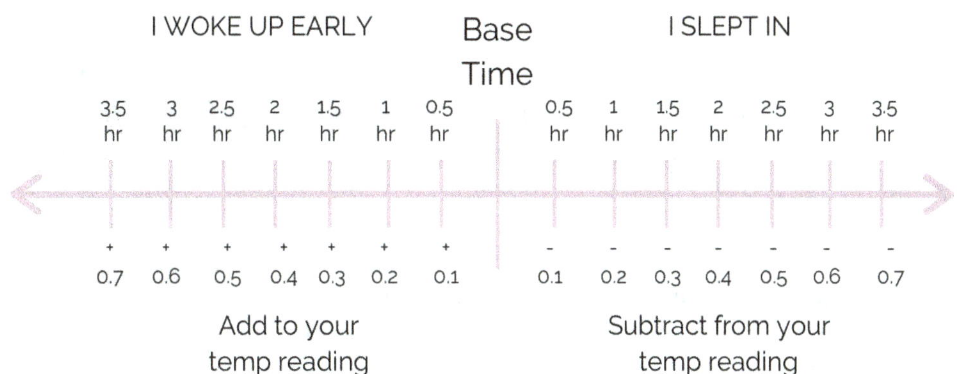

Practice Examples:

Check your answers at the end of this book

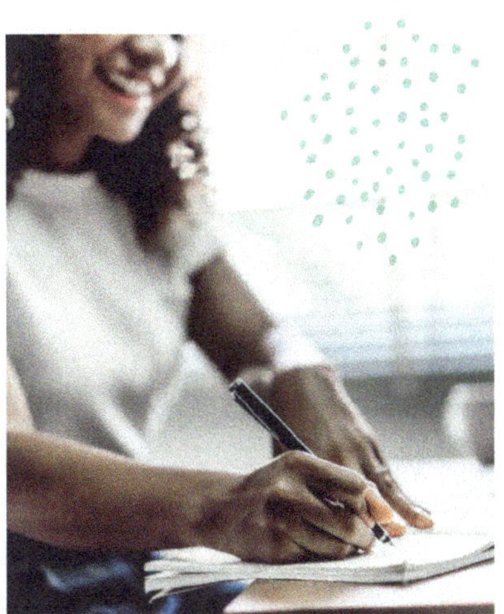

Example 1

Base Time: 7:00 AM
Wake up time: 8:00 AM
Her thermometer read: 97.4°
She will chart: ___________

Example 2

Base Time: 7:00 AM
Wake up time: 8:30 AM
Her thermometer read: 97.8°
She will chart: ___________

Example 3

Base Time: 7:00 AM
Wake up time: 6:30 AM
Her thermometer read: 97.7°
She will chart: ___________

Example 4

Base Time: 7:00 AM
Wake up time: 5:00 AM
Her thermometer read: 97.1°
She will chart: ___________

LH TESTS: What are they?

At-home LH Tests can go by many different names:

- Ovulation Predictor Kits
- Ovulation Tests
- LH Strips

Much like thermometers, there can be a wide range of test options depending on how much money you want to spend, but the fact is that more expensive tests don't always get you the best results! All of these tests are looking for the same basic thing: the presence of Luteinizing Hormone (LH) in your urine. LH is the pituitary hormone which surges right before ovulation, so a positive result usually tells us that ovulation will happen within the next few days. When combined with cervical fluid and/or temperatures, LH tests can be a very helpful tool to have on our charts.

HOW TO USE LH TESTS

Always follow the instructions for the specific brand you are using. LH is a hormone which tends to surge midday, so the best chance to catch a positive reading is by using a test late in the morning or in the early afternoon. To take the test, you will need to collect a small sample of urine into a cup. Your test stick will have a dipping end: do not submerge the stick into the urine past the maximum dipping line. Your instructions will tell you how long you should dip the stick in the sample and how many minutes to wait before reading the test.

Prior to testing, you will probably want to limit your water intake and make sure that you have a 2-3 hour hold with your urine in order to get the best concentration. If it's not feasible for you to take a test in the middle of the day, then using your first morning urine (FMU) is usually alright. If you discover after a few cycles that you're missing your LH surge or getting too many positive results with FMU, it is likely that you will need to change your testing time.

Advice can vary about when to start testing with LH strips. As you gather more data about your cycles, you could choose to save time and money by beginning your testing four days prior to your earliest previous positive LH test. So if the earliest cycle day you saw a positive result was on day 12, you would begin testing on day 8. As you start charting, it is easiest to just begin LH testing the day after your period has ended. Once you have started testing, you will need to test every day until you can verify that ovulation has passed.

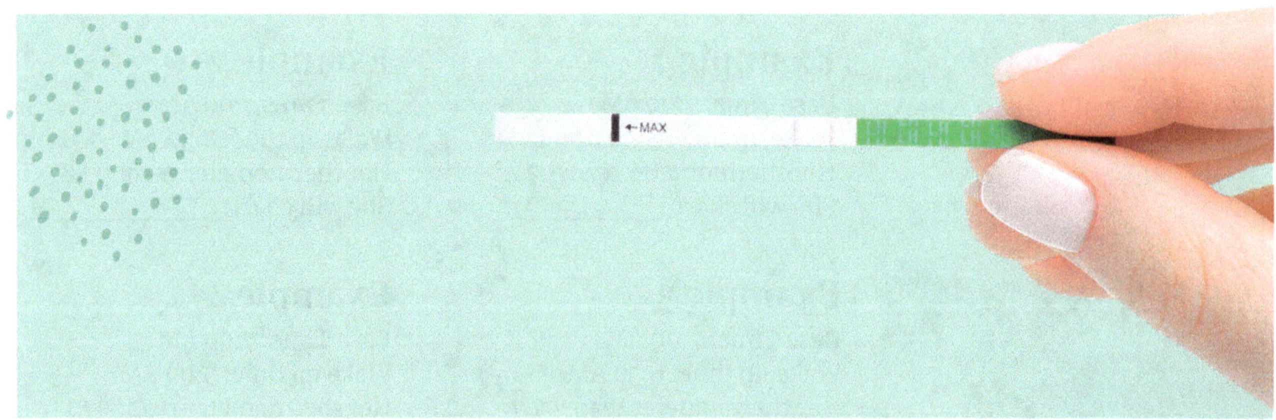

LH TESTS: Recording on a Chart

HOW TO READ LH TESTS

An LH Test should always show you a control line which you will use as a comparison point for your test line. If your test line is absent or lighter than the control line, then the result is negative. If your test line is the same shade or darker than the control line, then the result is positive. If the control line is absent, the result is invalid.

On your chart, record your LH results with a negative (-) or positive (+) interpretation.

If you need assistance reading an LH test, you can take a photo of the test and put it into a specific app for interpretation. A simple search for "free LH test tracker app" will yield many options. In some cases, apps will give you a quantitative number reading along with an interpretation of whether the app thinks the LH test is low, high, or peak value. This is actually more information than most women need for cycle charting, so regardless of those interpretations, I still recommend charting a simple negative or positive result on your chart. If you are given a quantitative reading, you'd be looking for a number value of 1.0 or higher to mark a positive result. Anything less than 1.0 is a negative result.

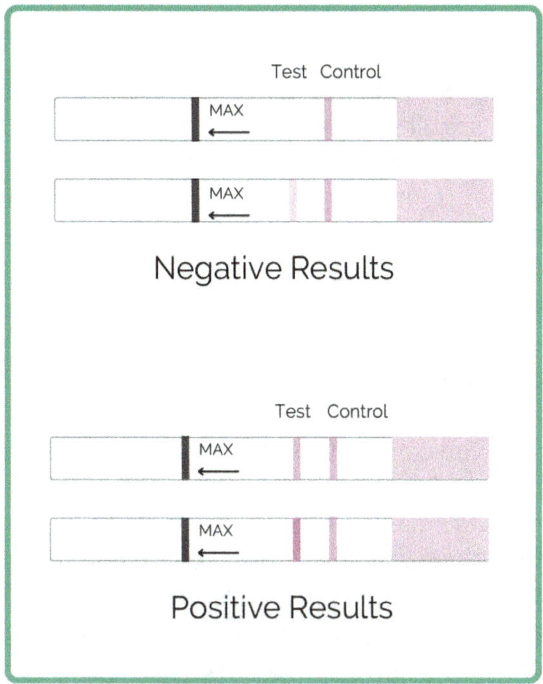

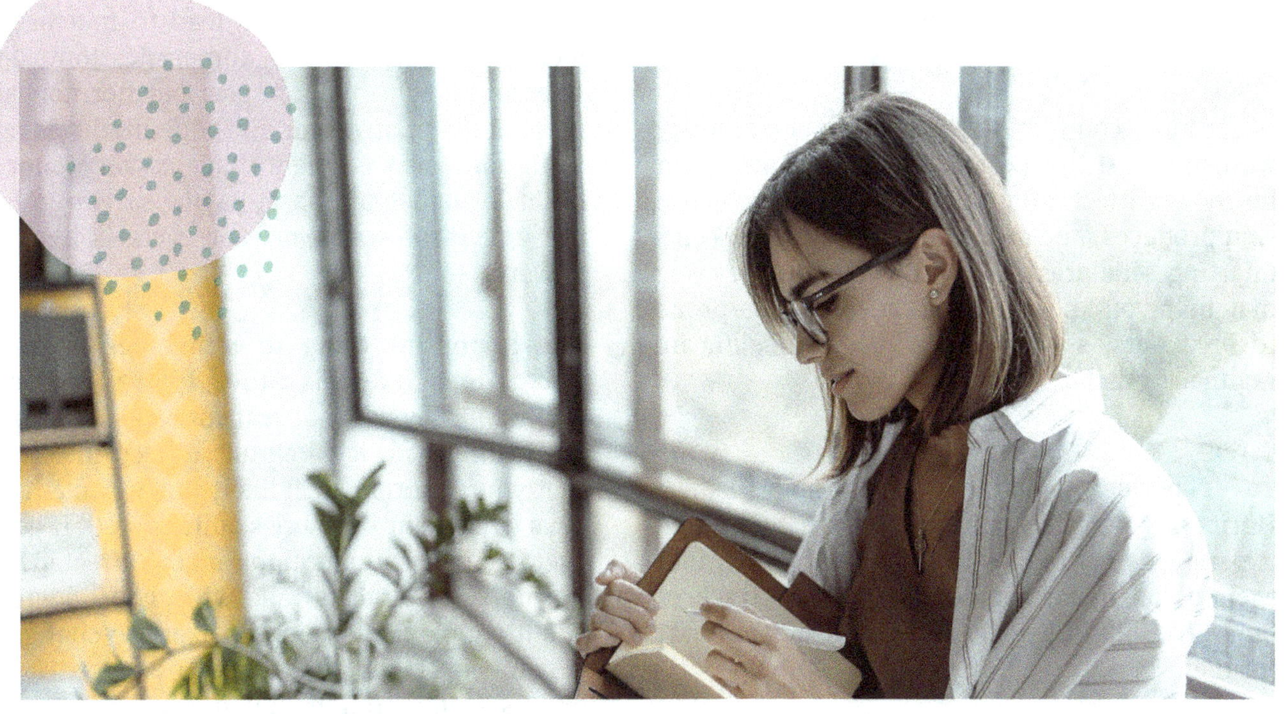

Using Custom Fields for Tracking

WHAT OTHER SIGNS CAN I TRACK?

As you get to know your cycles, you may notice more changes than just fertility biomarkers. Our fluctuating hormones affect many aspects of our lives, creating a cyclical **infradian rhythm** on top of our regular circadian (daily) rhythm. The paper chart includes one line for custom tracking, but many apps will offer custom fields or note options to help you keep track of other things related to your cycle. Here are some common things women may choose to put on a chart:

HEADACHES

Some women experience hormonal headaches. If you are someone who gets lots of headaches, charting headaches and cycles can help your doctor figure out if they have hormonal patterns, or if they are likely caused by things other than fluctuating hormones.

EXERCISE

Everyone has different exercise goals to maintain a healthy lifestyle. If you met your goals for the day, you can mark it on your chart. Over time, you may notice certain patterns emerging about your exercise habits throughout the cycle: you may find that a type of exercise is easier during one part of the cycle than another. There are many emerging resources on cycle syncing your exercise routines for women, so you might consider switching up your exercise regimen to match the phase of the cycle you are in!

ACNE

While more common in the teenage years, many women will still experience hormonal acne. Our hormones affect inflammation, how much oil our skin produces, and even the activity of skin cells. Charting acne presentation throughout the cycle may help you know the key times you are prone to breakouts, so you can adjust your skincare regimen or diet accordingly.

BOWEL MOVEMENTS

Yes, "period poops" are a thing, ladies! Hormones can affect our bowels, so many women experience fluctuations in their stool throughout their cycle. If you would like to keep track of bowel irregularities, you can also use your chart for that.

MOODS

Changes in hormones can affect our emotions, and mental health should never be dismissed or neglected because it is "hormonal." By tracking our moods, we can better understand our reactions and energy levels on a daily and cyclical basis.

For example, when estrogen is high and "in charge," we tend to feel more energetic and happier. When progesterone is "in charge," we tend to feel quieter and more introspective. At the end of the cycle, our hormones all drop as we reset for the next cycle. This drop in hormones may cause some women to feel sad or like their emotions are stronger than normal, leading to PMS or PMDD.

Stress is also a mood we should pay attention to: certain hormones may lead to increased feelings of stress, but sometimes outside stressors may actually impact our hormones! If we are very stressed, our body might delay ovulation, or we might have a very short follicular or luteal phase. Paying attention to the effects of stress on our cycle is also a powerful tool.

The important thing to remember is that fluctuations like this are a typical part of cycling. They will not last forever, so if you are feeling bad, it's helpful to keep in mind that your emotions will likely change in a few days when your hormones shift as well. If you ever feel like your emotions are too affected by hormones, you can talk with your doctor about supplements, diet, or exercise changes which could help balance estrogen and progesterone throughout your cycle.

Tips for Building Charting Habits

Picking up the habit of cycle charting is not easy! It requires the user to not only learn all of the different biomarkers, techniques, and interpretation skills: it is something that can significantly impact your daily routine. At first, it may seem like a huge burden to try to incorporate charting into your life; but once charting becomes an ingrained habit, it will likely feel much less burdensome, and aspects of it may even provide new opportunities for you to think about and appreciate the hard (often invisible) work that your female body does!

In order to help you build this habit, here are a few tips I can offer after nearly a decade of coaching:

CERVICAL FLUID

Because this biomarker requires consistent monitoring throughout the day, it can be one of the more difficult habits to develop. If you find yourself forgetting to make observations or not being able to remember your observations throughout the day, try these tricks:

- At the beginning of the day, put three bracelets or different colored hair ties on your wrist. As you do this, tell yourself: "These are to help me remember to track fluid." When you go to the bathroom, you can move the bracelets around (either by switching wrists or by changing the order) to signify which category of fluid you observed.
- Take your phone into the bathroom with you and have an image of the category chart handy for reference. Use the chart to identify your fluid category and put it into a note on your phone or directly into your app.
- Once you're confident identifying peak-type fluid, cut yourself some slack with observations! A peak-type fluid observation means that the day will be categorized that way regardless of what else you see throughout the day. So if your first observation of the day is peak-type, mark that on your chart and move on with your day. Note, however, that if you're the sort of personality which will have a hard time being consistent after a time of laxity, this approach is not recommended!

TEMPERATURE

- Always keep your thermometer by your bedside to avoid losing it, and remember to remove the thermometer from the bed when you're done temping. Many thermometers have gone missing or gone through the wash because they have been lost in blankets. Keep a separate thermometer around for fever checks, because once something "wanders off," it can be hard to find!
- If you regularly hit snooze a couple of times, be sure you are consistent with which alarm is your base time. If you prefer to sleep in and are able to fall back asleep quickly, then set an alarm at a consistent time to take your temp and then just go back to bed. If you're totally irregular and unpredictable, or you're the type of person who jumps out of bed and can't stay still, then perhaps a wearable is better for you!

LH TESTS

- Avoid running out of tests by checking on your stash within the first few days of your period. If it's easiest to remember, just tell yourself that the first day of your period is "supply day."
- Set a reminder or an alert on your phone for the day before you need to start testing with LH tests. Make sure your cup and LH test are already set up in your bathroom or packed in your bag for the day.

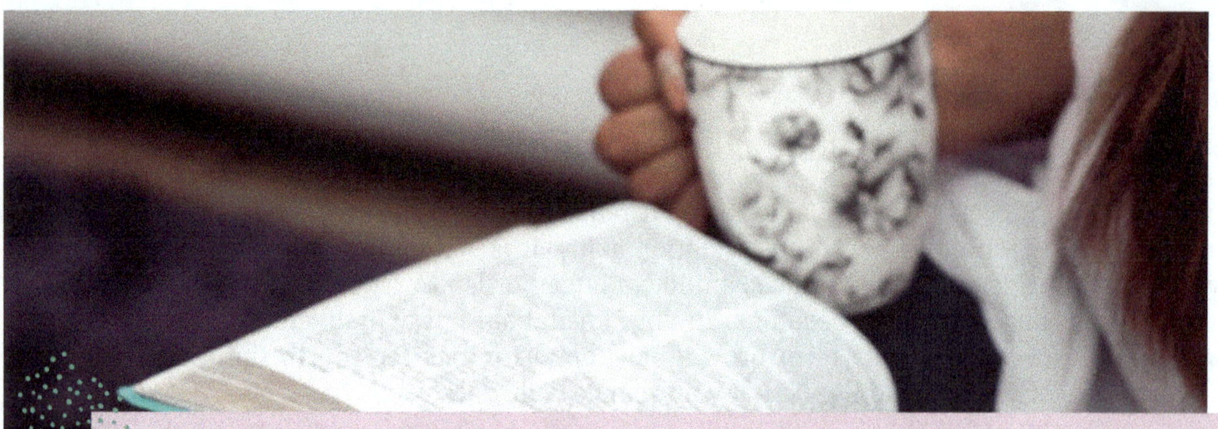

Reflection/Discussion Questions

Before we go on to learn about chart interpretations, let us take time to reflect on the invitation we have received, through cycle charting, to learn about and appreciate the unique design of the female body. Let us also think about questions or concerns we have with starting this new practice of charting:

- Does learning about this make me think differently about God's design of my body? If so, what is different? What new questions does it bring up for me?
- Men do not have this same window into their health and reproductive function. What are the positives to having this information? What could be some of the negatives?
- When have I successfully built new, healthy habits into my life? What were the key factors to my success? How can I incorporate those into my desire to learn more about my body?
- What additional support do I think I might need in order to succeed with this new practice of charting?

"As every woman's cycle is a little different, tracking your cycle can help you identify your own unique rhythms.... Over time, this information becomes a personal health compass—giving you important information not only about whether your cycle and related hormones are working optimally but if other signs and symptoms are cycle-related. Understanding your personal cycle can therefore be a tremendous source of health empowerment."

–Dr Aviva Romm

"For we are his handiwork, created in Christ Jesus for the good works that God has prepared in advance, that we should live in them."

–Ephesians 2:10

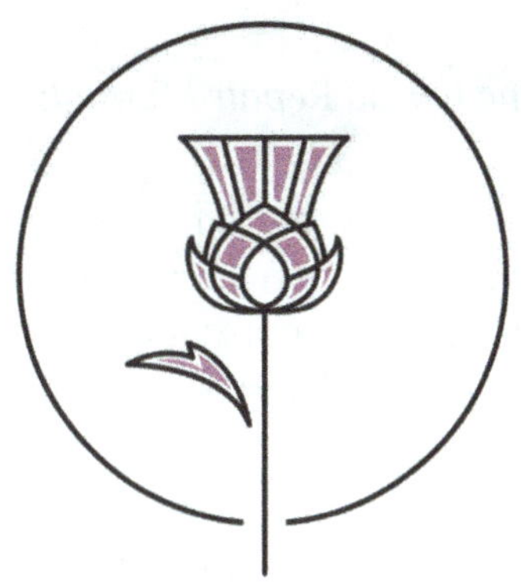

WHAT
CAN CHARTING TELL ME?

Why We Look for Ovulation

Before we learn how to interpret all of this information on our charts, let's spend a little bit of time talking about the value of doing all of this work in the first place. Why do we want to look for ovulation?

Lara Briden, ND, states in her book *The Period Repair Manual:*

> Ovulation is well-recognized for its role in reproduction; however, since regular ovulation is only possible when your endocrine system and reproductive system are functioning normally, an irregular or abnormal cycle is an early warning sign of an underlying health problem.

When women are taught how to observe their menstrual cycles to look specifically for ovulation, we are equipped with a powerful tool for understanding our overall health. The unique patterns of our menstrual cycle are a way that our body can *communicate* to us when something is wrong, or at least requires attention.

But why, specifically, ovulation? Because to put it simply: ovulation is the main event of the cycle. Without ovulation, there's no division of cycle phases. **Without ovulation, there is no period.**

But if you're still having bleeds ... what could be going on?

When a bleed is not preceded by ovulation, we call it "anovulatory," and there are a few different types:

Anovulatory bleeds can naturally happen when an egg is significantly delayed in being released. When that happens, estrogen either doesn't have the ability to remain high enough to keep sustaining the endometrial lining (in which case the lining sloughs off) or it works basically unchecked by progesterone and produces lining to such an abundant extent that some begins to slough off anyway. In either case, you can see a bleed which might look convincingly like a period, except for the fact that it wasn't preceded by ovulation.

Additionally, many women around the world are routinely having a different sort of anovulatory bleed, which is a progesterone withdrawal bleed. The most common form of this is experienced under the influence of artificial birth control hormones. The way many progesterone-based options work is to provide a steady level of progesterone for a certain amount of time, then to withdraw that progesterone support through sugar pills or temporary removal of the device, causing a bleed which mimics a period; but because it was not preceded by a follicular phase which resulted in ovulation, these bleeds are not true period bleeds. Progesterone withdrawal bleeds may also be used therapeutically for some women to ensure that excess endometrial lining is not retained on a regular basis.

If you are on any sort of treatment plan which includes hormones, it's a good idea to check in with your doctor to understand what impact that may have on your ability to chart your cycles naturally.

Uncovering Anovulatory Bleeds

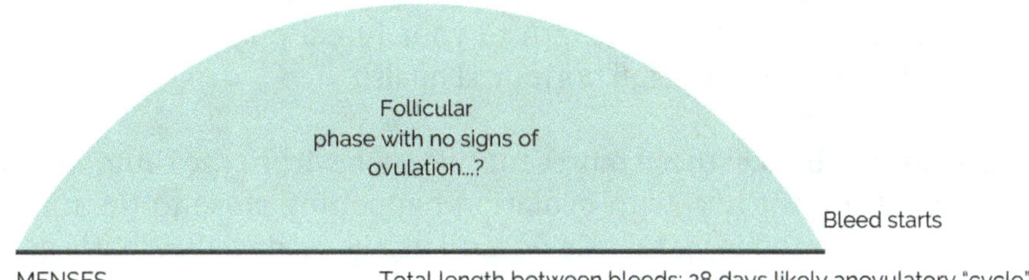

So, the first benefit of looking for ovulation is to just know if you're actually having a regular period bleed, and therefore are actually cycling in a normal and healthy way. You'd be able to identify this on a chart because period (ovulatory) bleeds are preceded by a build-up of peak-type fluid, a positive LH, and/or a discernible shift in temperature. If you do not see these things within about 10-16 days before a bleed, it's likely that your bleed could be anovulatory.

Why does this matter? Depending on your stage of life, anovulatory bleeds may not be a particular concern. They are fairly common in the first 3-5 years of cycling as our body learns how to put together all the necessary components of a cycle, and they increase again in frequency as we approach menopause. Certain medical conditions do make anovulatory bleeds more common, so the good news is that if you are charting for ovulation, you can learn to identify when you might be having these anovulatory bleeds and bring it to your doctor's attention.

CHARTING ANOVULATORY BLEEDS:
If you experience a bleed which was not preceded by any of the signs of ovulation we discussed:

- APP- mark the bleed and continue with the same cycle.
- PAPER- start a new chart so you don't run out of room. Title your charts as if they were a pair. For example: Old chart was Cycle #6, so you mark it as #6A. New chart is #6B.

If you are experiencing many bleeds which do not seem to have signs of ovulation, you can check with your doctor to see if there is a reason why you might be having hormonal bleeds which are not true periods. Think about whether you've had:

- change in diet (especially within the past three months)
- change in exercise
- weight loss or gain
- increased stress levels

...or anything else which might impact your body's ability to cycle.

Also pay attention to an increase in headaches, cramping, or other physical signs of discomfort which could help your doctor pinpoint the issue.

There are many reasons why a healthy woman may sometimes experience an anovulatory bleed. But if they become common, it is always a good idea to check things out.

Identifying Phase Consistency

Another benefit of charting for ovulation is that you can check to **see if your luteal phase is relatively consistent.** A predicable length to your luteal phase, even if your cycles are varying in length, is a good indicator of overall hormonal health.

Look at the examples below: these represent two cycles from the same woman. The first represents a typical cycle pattern for her, with ovulation happening close to the middle of the overall cycle. But one month, her period is "late" and doesn't arrive on day 28. What's going on?

By tracking our cycles to look for ovulation, we can actually know that in the second instance, her period isn't "late." She didn't see signs of ovulation until Day 22, which was much later than her typical Day 14. This is because our follicular phase is much more susceptible to variation than our luteal phase. Our bodies are very smart, and even though we cannot have total control over when ovulation happens, our bodies can *temporarily delay* ovulation if it seems like the circumstances aren't quite the right time for a pregnancy (or, in severe cases, shut it down altogether). Illness, stress, or other similar factors may mean that our follicular phase is lengthened due to delayed ovulation, but our luteal phase should remain fairly predictable. So after confirming ovulation has happened, we should have a predictable amount of time before our period starts.

Knowing this and being able to observe it in our body will eliminate moments of panic when we think our period is late, but it will also enable us to see if our luteal phase is actually fairly consistent, which is a good indicator of overall hormonal health, even if we do see some variation in our follicular phase from time to time.

TYPICAL OVULATION- EXAMPLE

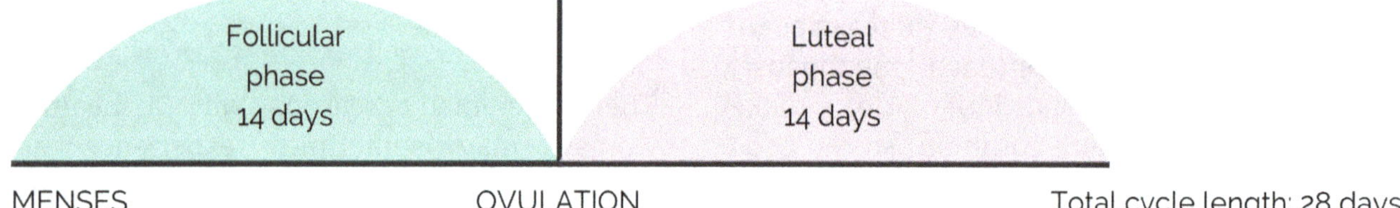

MENSES OVULATION Total cycle length: 28 days

DELAYED OVULATION- EXAMPLE

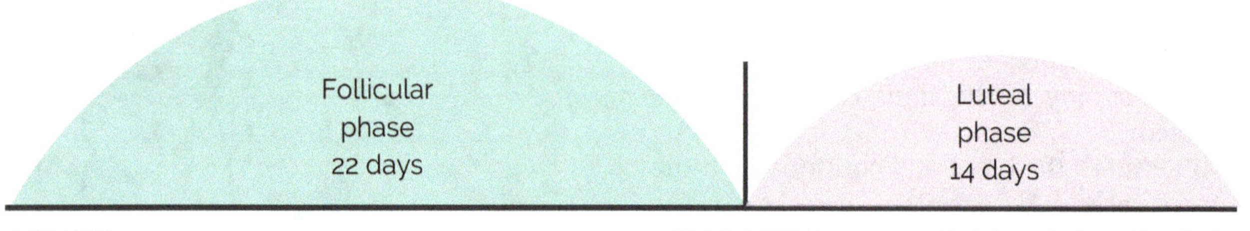

MENSES OVULATION Total cycle length: 36 days

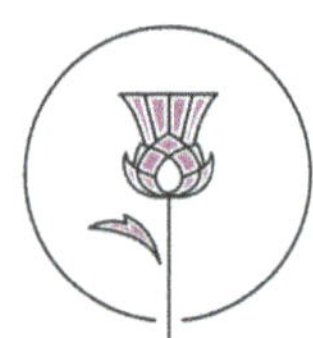

Note that in these examples we have a fictional world in which she can know the exact day she ovulated— a consistent luteal phase for you will likely be a small range (e.g., 12-14 days long) after you are able to verify that ovulation has passed.

Relative Lengths of Follicular and Luteal Phases

Another thing we can learn from charting for ovulation is that **not all cycles are the same**—even if they are the same length! Learning to identify ovulation means we can see some interesting things in cycles which we would NOT see if we were just looking at bleeds and lengths. Take a look at the examples below, all from different women who all experienced bleeds 28 days apart.

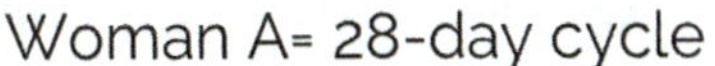

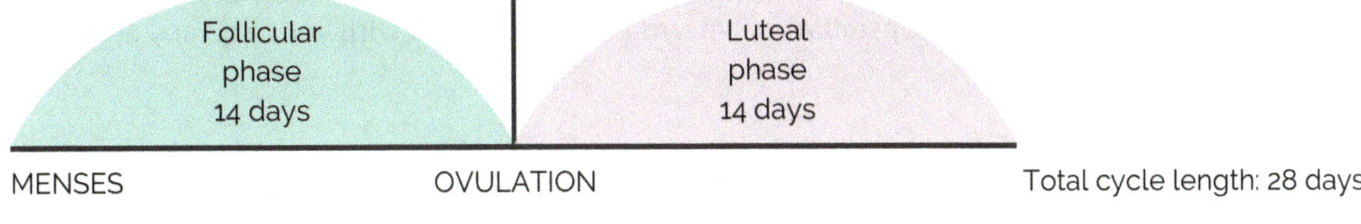

Woman B= 28-day cycle

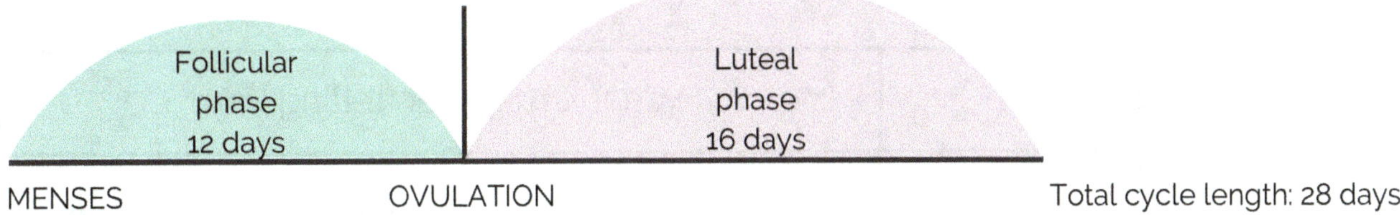

Woman C= 28-day cycle

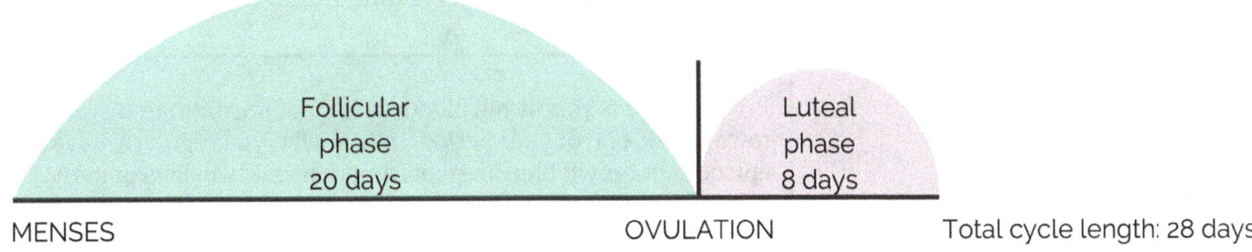

Woman D= 28-day cycle?

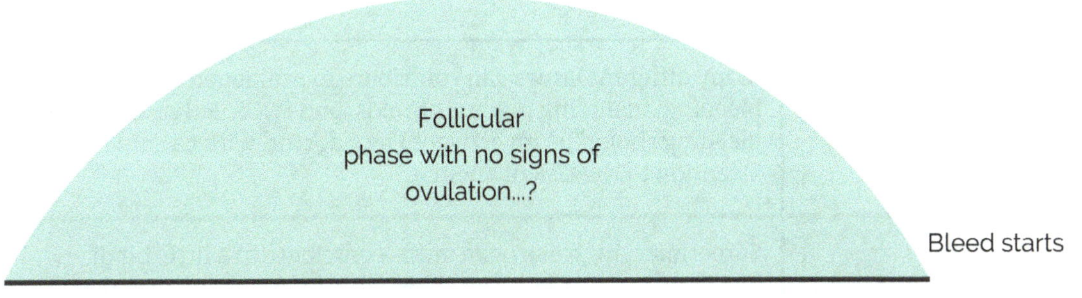

MENSES

Total length between bleeds: 28 days
likely anovulatory "cycle"

Common Issues to Spot on Charts

Learning how to observe and chart your cycle is not going to be a magic key which suddenly unlocks the answer to every health issue you've ever experienced; however, certain things may appear on your charts which—in conjunction with other symptoms and under guidance from your doctor—can provide additional information to help pinpoint some health issues. In the following pages, we'll discuss some common things our biomarkers may tell us about our cycles and overall health. **Please note that this section is not going to cover ALL health issues related to fertility and cycles, nor is it meant to be a substitute for consultation and diagnosis with your healthcare team!** Diagnosis cannot be done with a single indicator or issue: it requires the assistance of a trained professional who can look at a "constellation" of symptoms and work with you to do any additional testing.

BLEEDING ISSUES

Women who track their periods may be aware of some general bleeding patterns, but are not really observing the same level of detail that experienced cycle charters are. When you start to pay attention to your biomarkers more, you may notice things about your bleeding patterns that completely eluded you before! Here are a few things you might keep an eye out for:

What you observe:	What it might be telling you:
Premenstrual Spotting Days of red spotting prior to the start of your period flow	Low progesterone can sometimes mean that a woman will have spotting prior to the onset of her period, because her *corpus luteum* is not producing sufficient hormones to sustain the uterine lining. Spotting for two or more days prior to a period could also be an indicator of endometriosis, or a sign of polyps.
Tail-End Brown Bleeding Days of brown spotting or bleeding at the end of your period	Brown blood is simply old blood, so it's not uncommon to see towards the end of your period. If, however, you regularly have episodes of brown bleeding/spotting that last two days or more, it could be a sign that your progesterone is low, because it isn't breaking down uterine lining and clearing it at the rate it should.
Short/Light Bleeds A bleed lasting fewer than three days, or consisting of less than 5 mL total	Brief or scant bleeding episodes could indicate low estrogen, or they could be a sign of anovulatory bleeding.
Long/Heavy Period A bleed lasting more than seven days, or consisting of more than 80 mL total	Many different issues can contribute to prolonged and/or heavy bleeding, including polyps, fibroids, and PCOS. Extended bleeding should be investigated by a doctor, with careful attention to the risk of anemia.
Mid-Cycle Bleeding Any bleeding episode which is not preceded by ovulation	Sometimes, high estrogen levels contribute to a little bit of bleeding around ovulation. This can be a perfectly normal occurrence for some women, but frequent bleeding episodes that are not menses can also indicate other health issues like infection.

Common Issues to Spot on Charts

FLUID ISSUES

Fluid patterns tend to be one of the more highly-variable indicators I see with clients, but in general we can say that healthy presentation is a build-up of Non-Peak type fluid following menses, the appearance of Peak Type fluid around ovulation, then a change back to Non-Peak type or even Dry days following ovulation. Take note of the following issues which are fairly common to see on charts related to fluid observations:

What you observe:	What it might be telling you:
Continuous Fluid You never feel like you have a dry day, or you feel like all your observations are peak-type	Excess estrogen may create ongoing fluid observations, including the persistence of stretchy fluid after ovulation. Another less common culprit is cervical ectropion, where fluid-secreting cells are found outside the cervix. This can cause persistent discharge that makes it difficult to observe normal fluid patterns.
Scant Fluid You find it hard to make external fluid observations because it doesn't seem like much fluid is there	Low estrogen could mean you don't produce enough high-quality fluid, or it could mean that you are simply dehydrated! I always suggest that my clients watch their water intake to see if that improves fluid presentation. High-powered antihistamines can sometimes also dry up fluid signs.
Signs of Infection Fishy, metallic, or yeasty odors; appearance changes to green, gray or white chunky	Once you become familiar with your personal fluid patterns, you'll immediately notice if your fluid begins to produce an odor or deviates from standard coloring. Many infections, including yeast or bacterial vaginosis, can be identified early when a woman knows how to observe her healthy patterns!
Multiple Fluid Patches You observe more than one patch of peak-type fluid in a cycle	Stress or illness can delay ovulation, creating a prolonged cycle which may have multiple peak-type fluid patches. Other conditions like PCOS can also present with more than one series of fluid build-up.

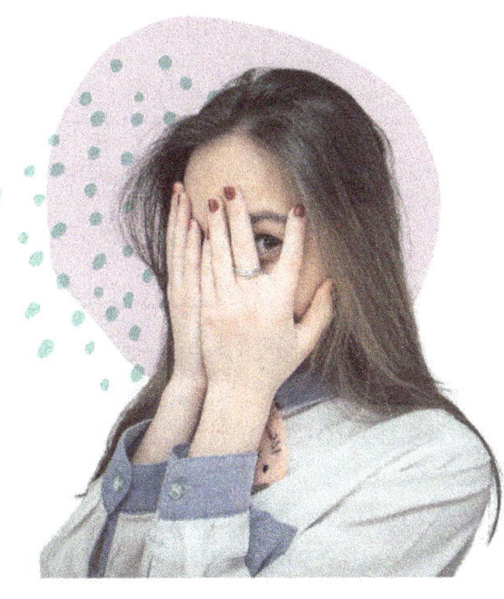

It is also worth noting that cervical fluid secretions are not the only thing we will observe coming out of our vagina! Arousal fluid is a lubricative type of fluid that is produced when we are sexually-aroused. If you notice gushes of fluid as a response to sexual stimuli, know that this is also healthy, normal, and **nothing to be embarrassed about**. Lubrication is the response of a woman's body to prepare her for more comfortable and pleasurable intercourse.

It is recommended that you pay attention to these responsive secretions and exclude them from your daily fluid observations. Specifically, you should wait at least sixty minutes after arousal to make a fluid observation.

Common Issues to Spot on Charts

TEMPERATURE ISSUES

Because temperatures track with progesterone, a lot of what they will tell us about health directly relates to how well our body is producing progesterone. In some cases, temperature issues will stem from poor technique or external variables beyond your control, so you can trouble-shoot a few issues by asking:

1. Am I consistent about taking my temperature at the same time each day?
2. Have I experienced any significant stressors, travel, or other lifestyle changes which are affecting my sleep (and therefore my ability to get reliable temps)?
3. Could my device be faulty or need a battery change?
4. Has my sleeping environment drastically changed?

Barring these issues, here are some key things to watch out for related to the temperature sign:

What you observe:	What it might be telling you:
Delayed Temperature Shift Your temperature rise starts three or more days after your other biomarkers have reached peak	This is what we colloquially call "sluggish progesterone," meaning that your *corpus luteum* is taking a while to produce enough progesterone.
Unsustained Temperature Shift Multiple temperatures dip below the coverline prior to the onset of menses	Fallback temperature patterns can similarly tell us that progesterone is not working at optimal levels in the luteal phase.
Insufficient Temperature Shift Fewer than ten days of high temperatures before the onset of menses	Short luteal phases mean that the body may not be producing progesterone long enough to allow adequate time for implantation, and might result in increased chance of early pregnancy loss.
Erratic Temperature Patterns You observe high variability of temperatures, especially prior to ovulation	It's possible that jumpy temperature patterns could be a sign of low estrogen, since estrogen works to stabilize temperatures prior to ovulation; but as long as you get a reliable set of low temperatures prior to a shift, it may not be an issue!
Prolonged Temperature Shift 16+ days of high temperatures	If pregnancy is not possible, then a temperature shift which lasts longer than 16 days may indicate a luteinized unruptured follicle (LUF) or the presence of an ovarian cyst.
Temps Don't Fit on the Chart Your temperature is too low or high to fit on the standard graph	Hypo- and hyper-thyroid issues can produce lower or higher than normal temperatures, respectively. This is not diagnostic in and of itself, but could be discussed with a doctor. Another thing to keep in mind is that thermometers are calibrated differently, and some wearable devices, especially, may have lower normal ranges of readings because they do not measure oral temps.

Common Issues to Spot on Charts

LH TESTING ISSUES

Unlike fluid and temperatures, LH testing is not looking at a secondary *effect* of the hormone in the body: we are looking at the urinary metabolites of that hormone itself. As long as you are following the testing techniques and recommendations for your specific brand, there are minimal issues we see with LH tests. As an instructor, I expect that at-home hormone monitoring will become increasingly detailed and we will likely see more research about these biomarkers. For now, a couple of simple things can be observed with these tests:

What you observe:	What it might be telling you:
No LH Surge You get a bleed, but never saw a positive LH test	If you didn't get a positive LH, it could mean that you are testing at a time which is not optimal for your body, or your urine is too diluted to get a good read. You can trouble-shoot this by following the instructions carefully for your specific brand. If this does not yield a change in results and you still are not seeing positive LH readings before a bleed (especially if you also don't see a temp rise!), it could mean that your bleeds are anovulatory.
Frequent LH Surges You get positives, but they are not followed by temperature shifts or bleeds. This may happen multiple times before you finally verify ovulation	PCOS is the primary culprit in this scenario, because women with PCOS tend to have a higher baseline level of LH and/or see frequent surges which do not result in ovulation.

TYPICAL CYCLE SUMMARY:

In general, the parameters below are considered to be key markers for an overall healthy cycle. If your cycle does **not** meet these parameters, it doesn't necessarily mean that there is anything wrong, but it is worth a conversation with your doctor just to check in:

Cycle Length	21-35 days (although 24 days is also commonly cited for low end), with fewer than 8 days of variation between consecutive cycles
Period Length	3-7 days with at least one day of moderate or heavy bleeding
Volume of Period Flow	5-80 mL total blood loss over the course of a period represents extreme ends of the range, but a more typical range is between 25-60 mL (about 2-4 tablespoons)
Luteal Phase	While the follicular phase can vary, the luteal phase should remain fairly consistent each cycle: ranging between 10-16 days

Journal Page

This section reviewed why ovulation is important to track in our cycles, and offered some key insights about what information different biomarkers may give us. Use this page to write out any questions you have about your cycles, and see if this can help you figure out which biomarkers you might like to track.

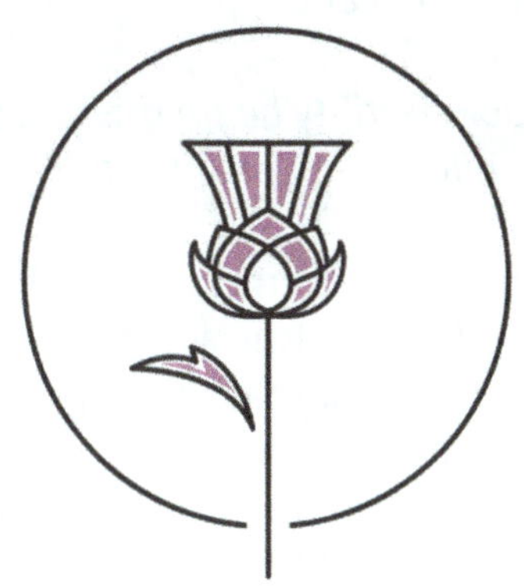

HOW TO
INTERPRET A CHART

Using a Chart to Identify Ovulation

Now that you know how to chart three different biomarkers of ovulation, and why that might be important, let's talk about how to use that information. When using a method of NFP, you will need to be able to determine two things with this data:

When does fertility begin this cycle; and
When does fertility end?

For our purposes, we will be answering a different question. Instead, we will be asking: when can I be certain that ovulation has passed? **We can't know the EXACT day of ovulation with current at-home techniques,** but we know that each biomarker happens within a certain window around ovulation, so the answer to that question might be different depending on which of the biomarkers you choose to incorporate. This guide will walk through each sign independently, and then talk about how to use them in various combinations together.

TO IDENTIFY OVULATION HAS PASSED BY INDIVIDUAL SIGN:

Cervical Fluid	BBT	LH Tests
Identify the Fluid Peak Day. Count 4 days after Fluid Peak Day.	Identify a temperature shift. Count 4 days of high temperatures.	Identify the LH Peak Day. Count 4 days after LH Peak Day.

TO IDENTIFY OVULATION HAS PASSED WITH COMBINATIONS:

3 SIGNS: Peak Day + 4 + 4 High Temps + Peak Day + 4

BBT + LH: 4 High Temps + Peak Day + 4

FLUID + BBT: Peak Day + 4 + 4 High Temps

FLUID + LH: Peak Day + 4 + Peak Day + 4

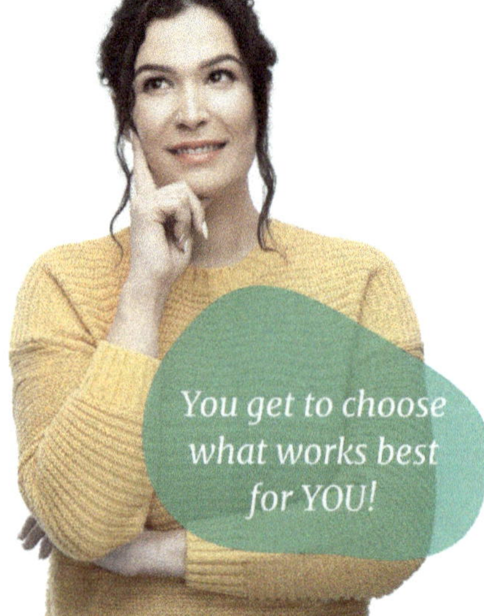

CERVICAL FLUID: Finding Peak Day

Around ovulation time, your body will make the Peak Type category of fluid as estrogen surges and works on those cervical crypts. So we'll check to see when it stops making this fluid, to let us know that ovulation has likely passed. For our purposes, **"Peak Day" will be defined as the last day of your most fertile sign,** which in the case of fluid is precisely that Peak Type category. So to identify it on your chart, you will look for the last day of fluid recorded with a peak type symbol, followed by 4 consecutive days which are either dry or non-peak type. This means that Peak Day can only be identified after it has occurred.

If you are using a paper chart, use the "Fluid Notations" line to mark Fluid Peak Day with a "☆" and number the four consecutive days after it.

What you're really looking for to identify Fluid Peak Day is a Peak Type category day followed by four consecutive not-Peak Type days, whether those are dry or non-peak categories. This will tell you that ovulation **has likely passed.**

EXAMPLE:
On your paper chart, the fluid key is:

O = dry day
⊖ = non-peak day
⊕ = peak type day

These six days of Peak Type category fluid could be called a **fluid patch,** which is a common thing to see leading up to ovulation. However, you may not get a clear patch like this: instead you could see a mixed pattern like: O, ⊖, ⊕, ⊕, ⊖, ⊖, ⊕, ⊕

After Peak Day, there can also be a lot of variation in fluid patterns, so don't worry if you have a mix of non-peak and dry days.

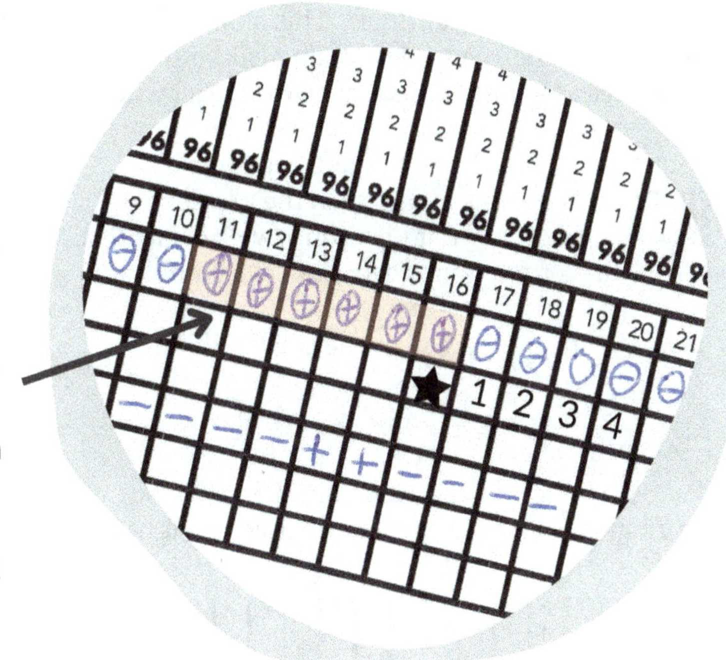

Why do we count 4 days?
Statistical observation shows that ovulation can happen within a window on either side of the cessation of peak-type fluid. Ovulation might occur *prior to* cessation/change in fluid, or it might occur *up to a few days afterwards.* So in order to have the highest degree of certainty about ovulation having occurred, we look for this particular pattern of four non-peak days after appearance of Peak Type fluid. For NFP methods, this count will vary slightly based on method and the particular characteristics included in their fluid categories.

BASAL BODY TEMPERATURE: Finding a Shift

A temperature shift shows us that progesterone is working, meaning that the follicle which had been developing within the ovary has already released its egg and become a *corpus luteum*. When we talk about temperature shifts, there are a few things to keep in mind:

1. It's all relative: everyone has a slightly different range that their pre-ovulation and post-ovulation temperatures will fall into. Additionally, thermometers can be calibrated differently. So for the most part, we aren't looking for your shift to reach a particular number on the graph. Every women doesn't have to hit 98.6 degrees to qualify! What we're looking for is a verified shift relative to YOUR unique pre-ovulatory temperatures.
2. Some women see shifts which are more drastic than others. You may find that your temperature shifts are very easy to see on a chart because there is a big jump (greater than .5 degrees) in your temperatures. But other women will see less dramatic shifts, and within certain parameters that can be perfectly healthy.

As you are beginning to learn this skill, you can always wait until the end of your cycle to retrospectively identify a temperature shift. Shifts are much easier to spot when you're able to see the context of the full cycle. Eventually, though, you'll probably want to learn how to identify a temperature shift "in real time." This skill will be necessary for using this information for family planning down the road, but it can also be helpful even for single women because you can use temperatures as a fairly reliable sign to predict when your period might arrive!

The temperature sign has a few different steps:

- **FIRST:** find 4 temps higher than the previous 6
- **SECOND:** calculate your Coverline *(we'll define that soon!)*
- **THIRD:** look for 4 temps over the Coverline

It's important to take these steps one at a time!

STEP ONE:

Go day by day across the chart and identify four consecutive temperatures which, as a set, are higher than the six temperatures that come right before them. This tells you that progesterone is working.

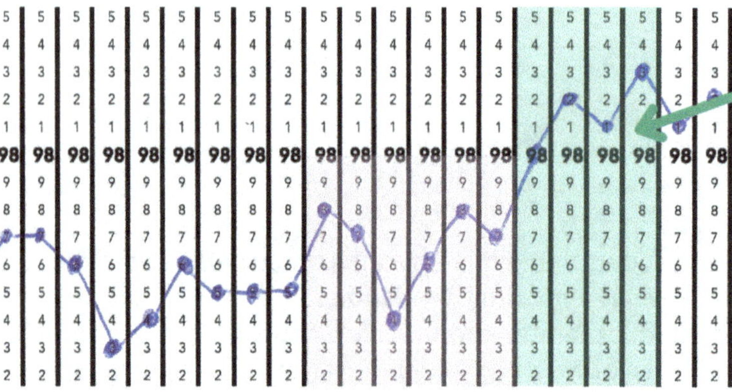

These four temperatures highlighted in green (98.0, 98.2, 98.1 and 98.3) are higher than the six that come before them, highlighted in purple to the left.

Note: it doesn't matter if the four temperatures are higher than each other! It only matters that they, as a group, are higher than the 6 days before.

BASAL BODY TEMPERATURE: Finding a Shift

STEP TWO:

Locate the highest temperature of the six low temperatures.
Draw a line across the chart 1/10th of a degree above this highest temperature. This is your **Coverline,** which is the dividing line between your low and your high temps.

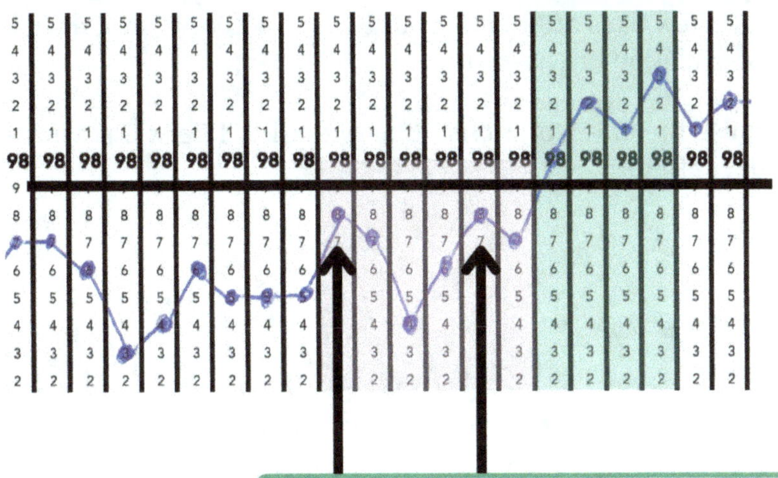

Note: when you are setting the Coverline, don't worry if there are temperatures earlier in your chart that might be on or above the line. You only need to look at the 6 temps which are right before your 4 high ones.

There were two temperature readings at 97.8 degrees in the set of low six. That is the highest number in the set, so your Coverline goes 1/10th of a degree above that at 97.9.

STEP THREE:

Number the first four temperatures **above** the line. Temps which are resting **on** the line don't count, but you don't have to redraw your line if this happens. You can just wait until you get 4 over the line. Once you do, this confirms for you that ovulation has passed! After you identify a shift, you can choose to stop charting temperature, or you can choose to keep charting and watch out for a temp that drops below your Coverline. This could be a signal that your period will start very soon!

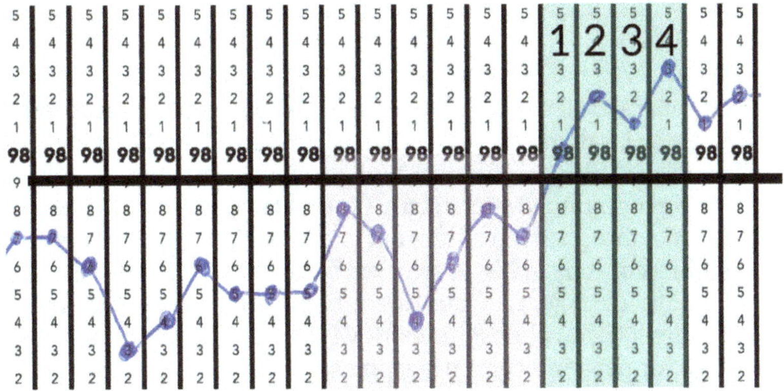

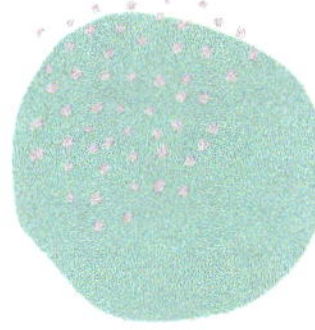

HELPFUL HINT!: Take it just a day at a time.

When you get that first 97.8 reading, you might think a shift is starting because it is higher than the 6 before it! You'd make a mental note to keep track of whether the next 3 days are also higher than the previous 6 ... which, in this case does not happen. So you just keep charting!

LH TESTS: Finding Peak Day

This is a very similar calculation to finding the Fluid Peak Day, but just looking at a different biomarker. Remember that **"Peak Day" is the last day of your most fertile sign,** which in the case of LH tests is going to be a positive reading. So to identify it on your chart, you will look for the last day of a positive reading, followed by 4 consecutive days of negative readings. Like Fluid Peak Day, this means that LH Peak Day can only be identified after the fact. Similarly, we know that ovulation can happen within a window of a few days after an LH surge, so we count out 4 days to have the highest degree of certainty that ovulation has passed.

If you are using a paper chart, use the "LH Notations" line to mark LH Peak Day with a "☆" and number the four consecutive days after it.

In this example, she has recorded two days of positive LH tests (OPKs) and the rest are negative. LH surges can vary in length, so it is possible that you could have two days like the example, or you may have a single day of positive. You could also have a slightly longer surge. Different NFP methods will vary on whether they count from a first positive LH or the last. For simplicity with this guide, keep testing and recording until you have FOUR full days of negative readings after a surge, no matter how long it was.

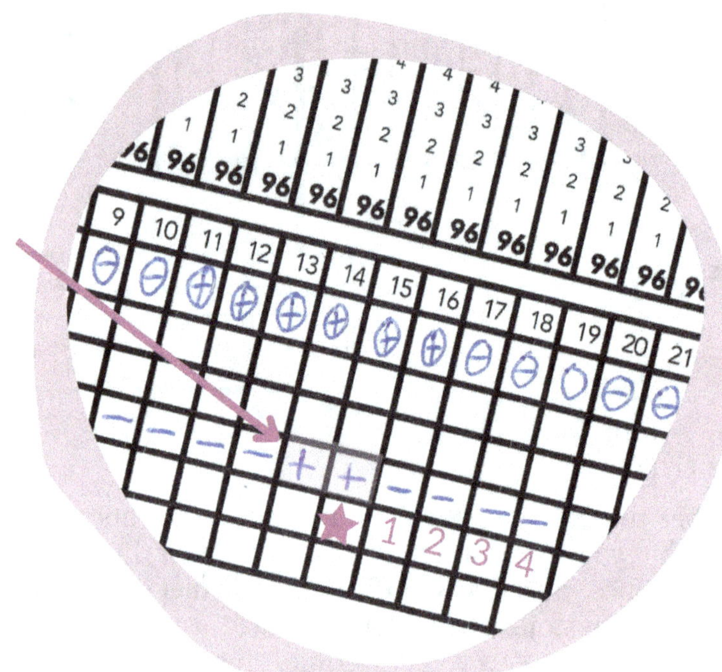

NOTE: APPS AND PEAK DAY

In general, I like that there are apps which can help us interpret some of these biomarkers, because it's sometimes good and even helpful to double check our own interpretations against something which has been programmed specifically for this task; however, I have seen apps want to interpret low, high, and peak readings on LH tests and they do so **inaccurately.** This is why our charting limits the LH notation to positive or negative, and identifies Peak Day as the last day of a positive. If you choose to work with an app which wants to give low, high, or peak interpretations, please make sure that you know how to verify if that "peak" interpretation is correct and can do this manual calculation for your own chart.

PRACTICE CHART 1: All Three Signs

Before we begin with practice charts, I think I should tell you that all of the data I am about to show you is completely fabricated. These sample charts are not exactly transcribed from real client charts, so if your cycles do not look like this or if your data collection is more sporadic, then please don't be concerned! Remember that real life is messier than these samples may show. That being said, these charts do represent the general patterns that I would be looking for as an instructor in healthy cycles, and it is possible for your charts to look like this once you are well-settled into the habit of charting and are confident with your data collection techniques.

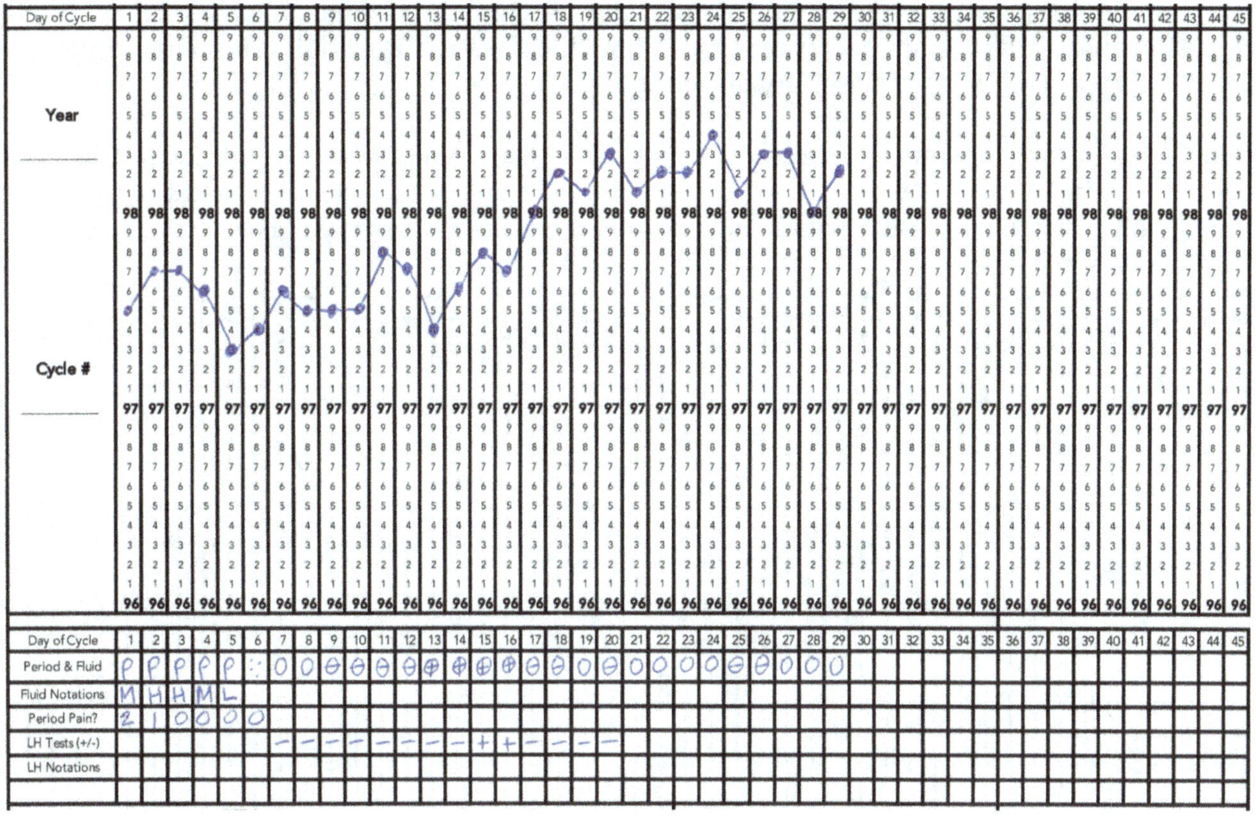

Now let's try to put this knowledge together to identify ovulation on a chart using all three biomarkers. With all three signs, you will know that ovulation has passed when you've been able to identify **FLUID PEAK DAY**, a **TEMP SHIFT**, and **LH PEAK DAY.**

We are looking at a completed chart, which is a different experience from working with a chart day-by-day as you are uncovering the data. As you are starting to chart, you could decide to wait until you finish a cycle to do any interpretations, so you'd be working with data more similarly to how it appears here.

A quick glance at this chart tell us that her cycle lasted 29 days. You can see that in the first part of her cycle, temps are comfortably below 98 degrees, and later in the chart they go a little bit above 98 degrees. You can also see that there was a patch of Peak Type fluid which appeared and then went away, and that this roughly corresponds to some positive readings on the LH tests.

PRACTICE CHART 1: All Three Signs

The first thing we need to do is look at the individual signs.

FLUID PEAK DAY

Looking at the Period & Fluid line of the chart, we can see that the first five days of this cycle were bleeding days. The sixth day was spotting, marking the tail end of her period. Days 7 and 8 were **Dry**, indicated by the empty circle. Starting on Day 9, she saw some **Non-Peak** type fluid so she marked the symbol of the circle with a horizontal line. The next few days had **Peak Type** observations, so she marked the symbol of the circle with both a horizontal and vertical bar (the + sign). Starting on Day 17, however, she stopped noticing the Peak Type fluid. Her observations on Day 17, 18, 19, and 20 were all either Dry or Non-Peak.

This means she now has enough information to identify **Fluid Peak Day,** since she had a Peak Type day on 16, which was followed by four days which were not Peak Type. She would mark a star underneath Day 16 in the "Fluid Notations" line, and then count out the four days afterwards.

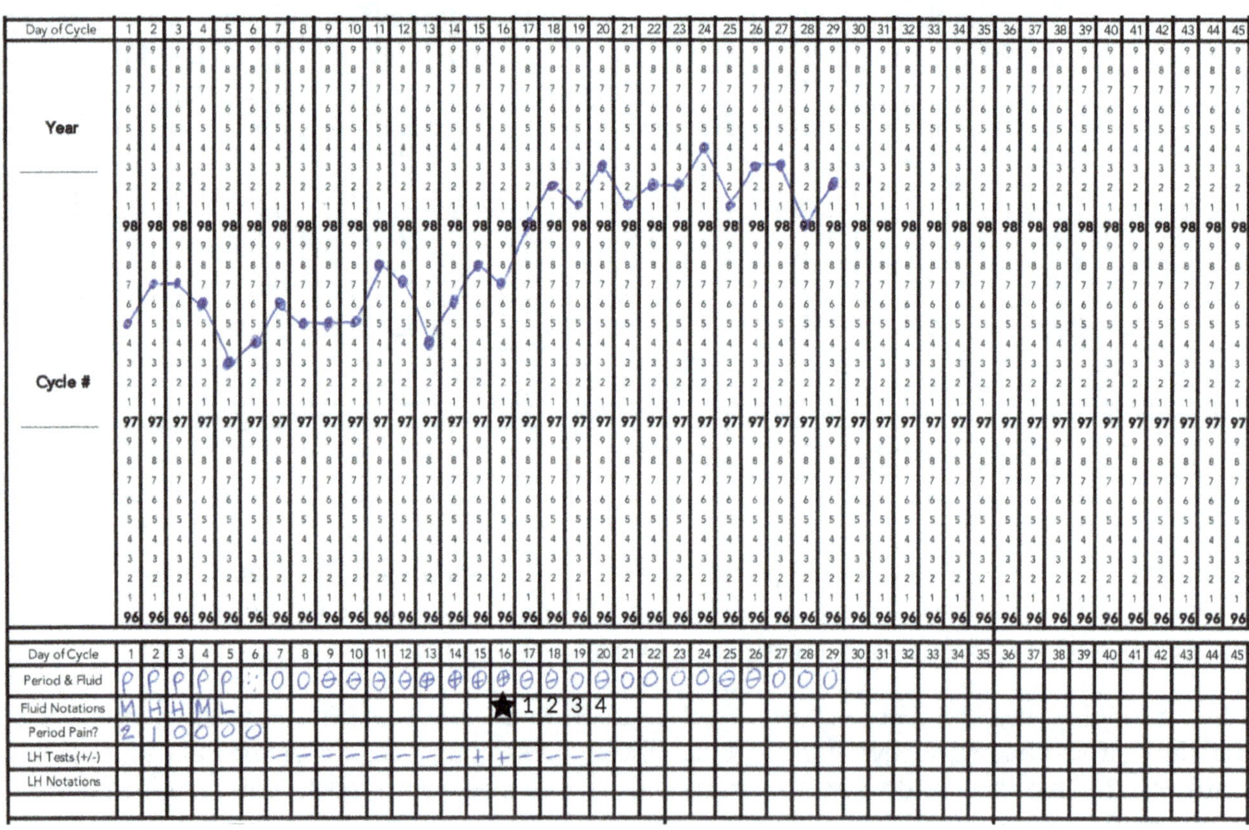

PRACTICE CHART 1: All Three Signs

TEMPERATURE SHIFT

There are three steps to identify a temperature shift.

- Look for 4 temperatures which, as a group, are higher than the 6 which come immediately before them.
- Identify the highest of the Low Six, and draw a Coverline 1/10th of a degree above it.
- Check to make sure that you have 4 temperatures above the Coverline.

We've actually done the calculation already on this chart with the sample given a few pages ago, but let's walk through it again:

Going day-by-day across this chart, the woman will want to ask herself: "Is today's temperature higher than the six before it?" The first time this happens is on Day 11, when she gets a reading of 97.8. On subsequent days, she would refer to days 10, 9, 8, 7, 6, and 5 as the possible set of six low temperatures if her shift were starting on Day 11. Although, let's be honest: she wouldn't think too hard about this because she is only having non-peak fluid signs!

So she sees that Day 12 is also higher than that group of low six, but then Day 13 is not. In this case, she will keep going with the chart. A few days later, on Day 17, she sees something that looks a little more convincing and which seems to line up with her fluid and LH observations as well. So now she's looking at days 16, 15, 14, 13, 12, and 11 as her potential Low Six. She sees that Day 18, 19, and 20 are all higher than those temps, so now she has 4 temps higher than the 6 before them.

Her Coverline goes at 97.9, since the highest value within the Low Six was 97.8 Days 17, 18, 19 and 20 are all ABOVE that line, so she has a verified shift!

Day of Cycle	1	2	3	4	5	6	7	8	9	10	11	12	13	14	15	16	17	18	19	20	21	22	23	24	25	26	27	28	29	30	31	32	33	34	35	36	37	38	39	40	41	42	43	44	45

Year

Cycle #

98

1 2 3 4

97

Low Six

96

Day of Cycle	1	2	3	4	5	6	7	8	9	10	11	12	13	14	15	16	17	18	19	20	21	22	23	24	25	26	27	28	29	30	31	32	33	34	35	36	37	38	39	40	41	42	43	44	45
Period & Fluid	P	P	P	P	P	[illegible]	O	O	⊖	⊖	⊖	⊕	⊕	⊕	⊕	⊕	⊖	⊖	O	⊖	O	O	O	O	⊖	⊖	O	O	O																
Fluid Notations	M	H	H	M	L											★	1	2	3	4																									
Period Pain?	2	1	0	0	0	0																																							
LH Tests (+/-)							–	–	–	–	–	–	–	–	+	+	–	–	–	–																									
LH Notations																																													

PRACTICE CHART 1: All Three Signs

LH PEAK DAY

The last step is to identify the LH Peak Day, which is the last day you see a positive (+) reading. To identify the LH Peak Day, we need to see a positive (+) followed by four consecutive days of negative (-) results.

On this chart, we see that she has two days of positive LH tests. She started testing on Day 7 when her period ended, and was consistent about testing every day. We will mark the last day of (+) reading as her LH Peak Day with a star, and then count out the four days afterwards to verify that ovulation has likely passed based on that sign.

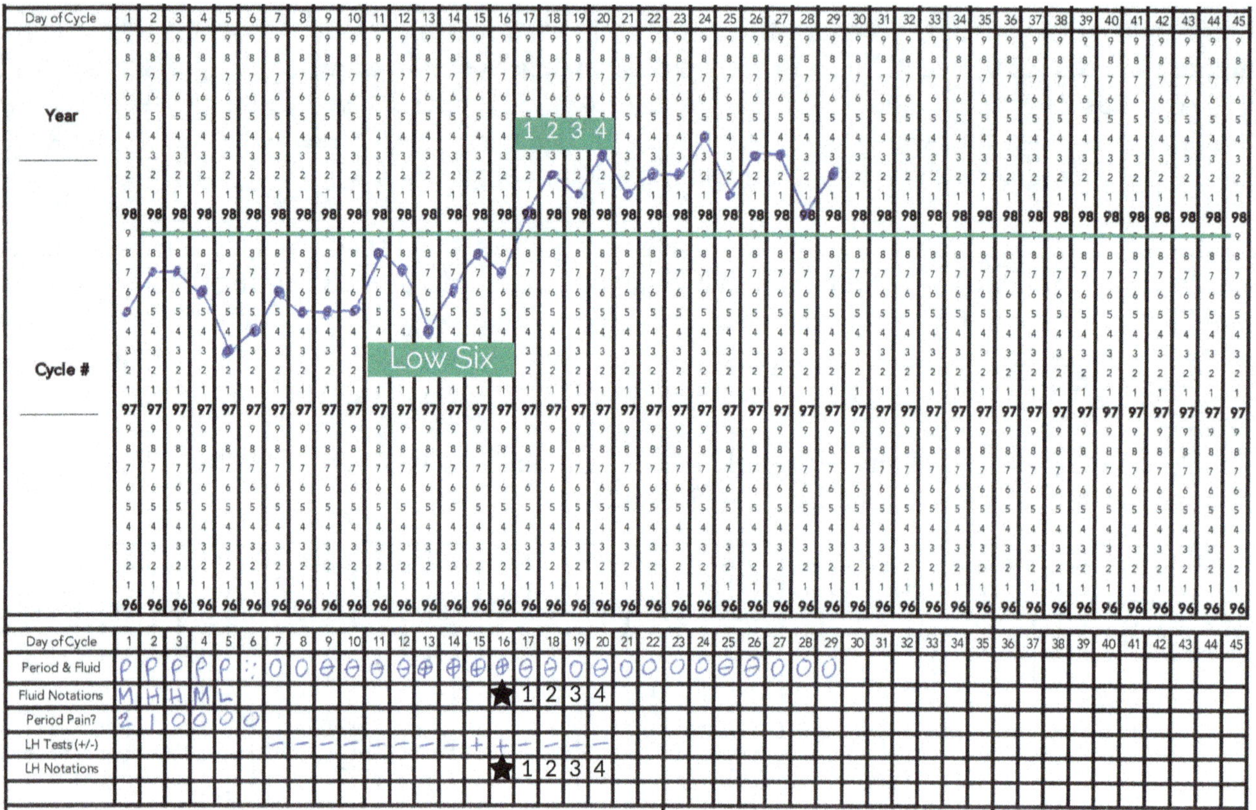

VERIFYING OVULATION HAS OCCURRED:

Now that we've computed all three of her signs, we let them "talk" to one another and see if they agree about when ovulation has passed.

FLUID PEAK was identified on Day 16, with end of count on Day 20.
TEMP SHIFT was identified starting on Day 17, with end of count on Day 20.
LH PEAK was identified on Day 16, with end of count on Day 20.

In this sample, **all three signs agree that ovulation has passed by Day 20**, since that is when all three of the counts are complete!

PRACTICE CHART 2 : All Three Signs, You Try!

Here's a similar sample chart for you to try.
Looking at the chart, see if you can figure out:

How many days long was this cycle? _______
How long did her period last? _______
How many days of Peak Type fluid did she see? _______

Date																																													
Day of Cycle	1	2	3	4	5	6	7	8	9	10	11	12	13	14	15	16	17	18	19	20	21	22	23	24	25	26	27	28	29	30	31	32	33	34	35	36	37	38	39	40	41	42	43	44	45
Year ______																																													
Cycle # ______																																													

Day of Cycle	1	2	3	4	5	6	7	8	9	10	11	12	13	14	15	16	17	18	19	20	21	22	23	24	25	26	27	28	29	30	31	32	33	34	35	36	37	38	39	40	41	42	43	44	45
Period & Fluid	P	P	P	P	P	O	O	⊖	⊖	⊖	⊖	⊖	⊕	⊕	⊕	⊕	⊕	⊕	⊖	⊖	⊖	O	O	O	O	O	O	O	O																
Fluid Notations	M	H	M	L	L																																								
Period Pain?																																													
LH Tests (+/-)								-	-	-	-	-	-	-	+	+	+	-	-	-	-																								
LH Notations																																													

Now try doing some calculations to verify that ovulation has passed.

What day was Fluid Peak? _______
When did her count after Fluid Peak end? _______
Where is the Coverline for temperatures? _______
What day was the start of her Temp Shift? _______
When did her count of high temps end? _______
What day was LH Peak? _______
When did her count after LH Peak end? _______
What day do all three signs verify ovulation has passed? _______

PRACTICE CHART 2 : All Three Signs, Answers

How many days long was this cycle? 29 days
How long did her period last? 5 days
How many days of Peak Type fluid did she see? 6 days

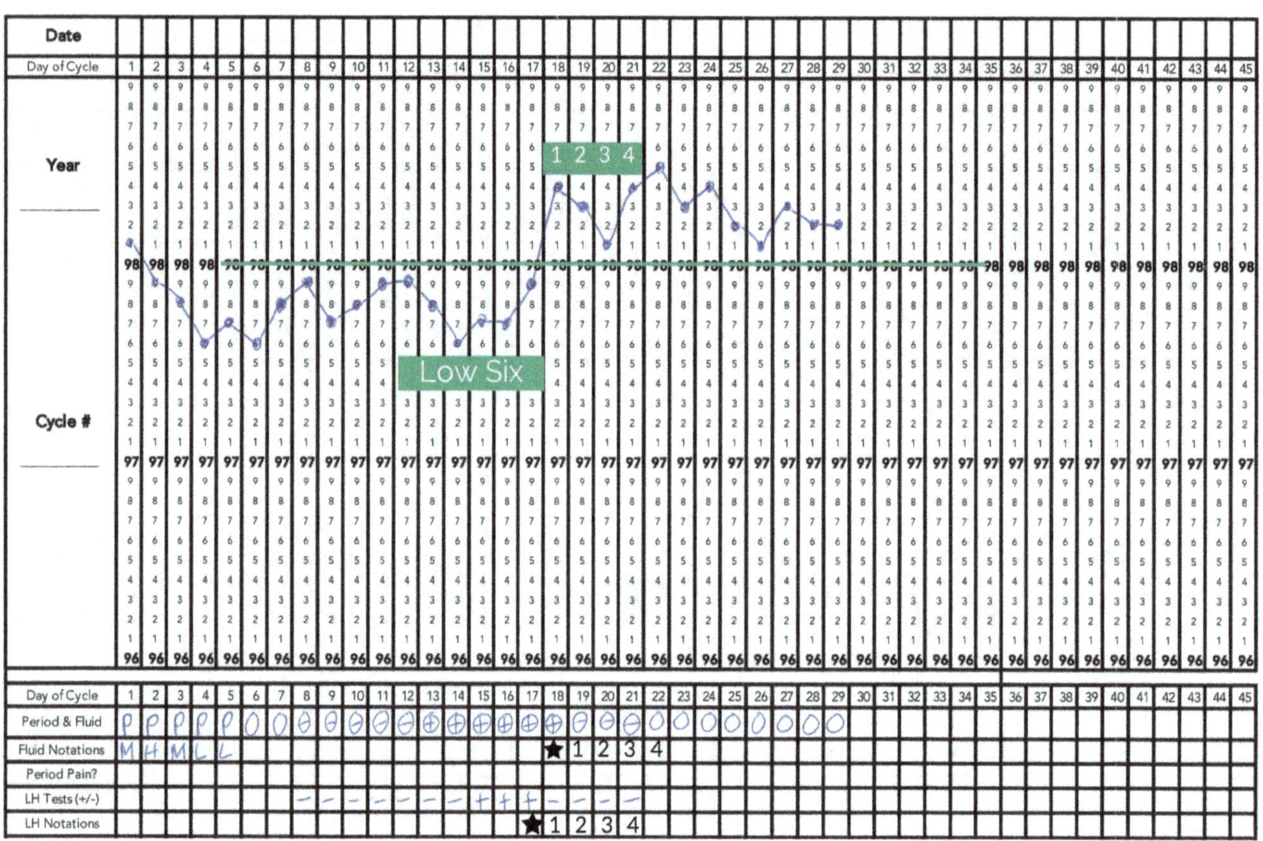

What day was Fluid Peak? Day 18
When did her count after Fluid Peak end? Day 22
Where is the Coverline for Temperatures? 98.0 degrees
What day was the start of her Temp Shift? Day 18
When did her count of high temps end? Day 21
What day was LH Peak? Day 17
When did her count after LH Peak end? Day21
What day do all three signs agree ovulation has passed? Day 22

NOTES:
The Coverline was placed at 98.0 because the highest value in the set of low six was 97.9.
All three signs agree that ovulation has passed by Day 22, because even though temps and LH agreed that Day 21 probably indicated ovulation had passed, the fluid count was not complete until Day 22.

PRACTICE CHART 3 : All Three Signs

Let's take a look at a chart where all three signs are being used, but something seems to be "off" with one of the signs.

We can easily see that this data set had a Fluid Peak Day on 16, and an LH Peak Day on 15. As we saw on the previous chart, it's possible for the signs to not line up exactly. Typically a difference of 1-2 days between any signs is not a concern at all, so we don't have to focus on that.

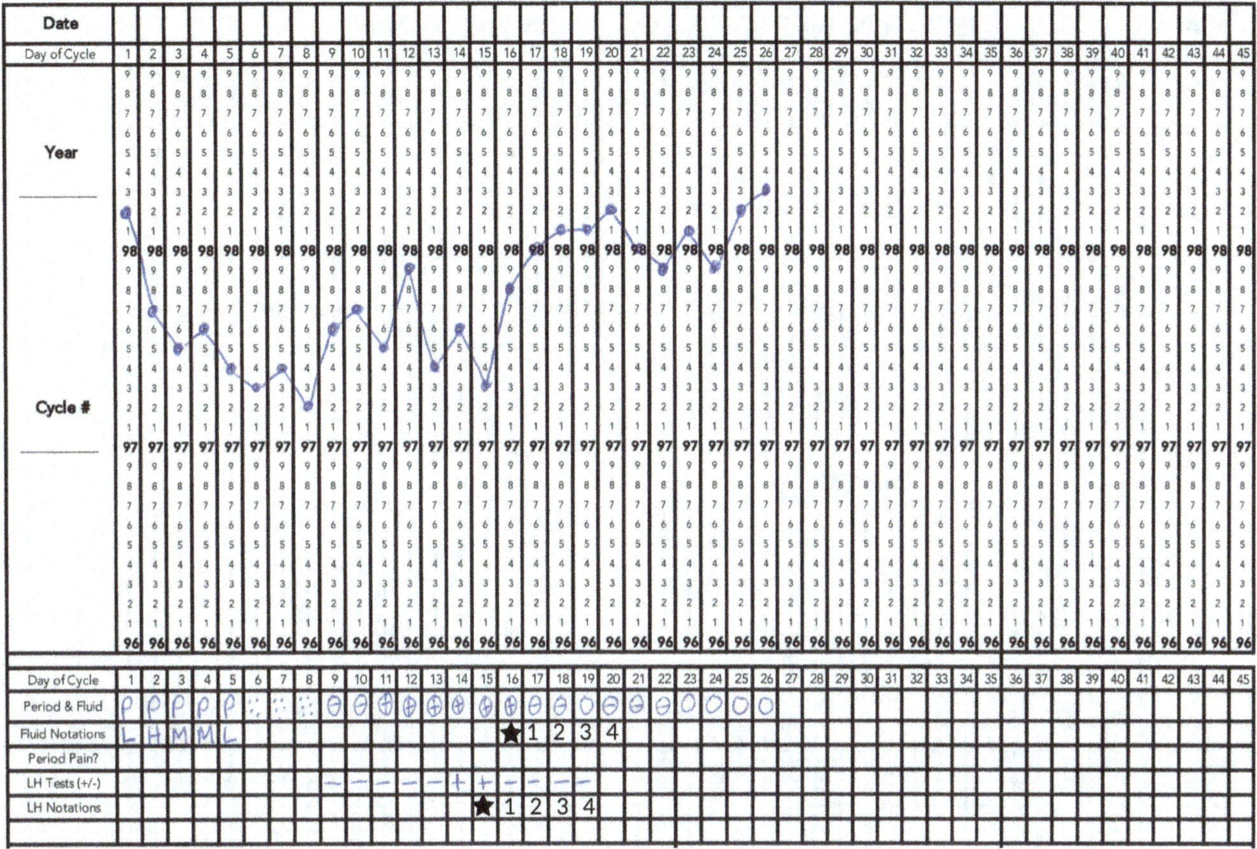

What I'd like to show you on this chart is an example of temperatures which don't quite seem to make sense. Going day by day across the chart, you see that Day 12 has a significantly elevated temperature. She has already started to see Peak Type fluid, but has not yet had an LH surge, so it's very unlikely this is an actual shift.

In this case, she would keep an eye on days 11, 10, 9, 8, 7, and 6 as her potential "Low Six" set and would see what happens the following few days. On Day 13, the temp goes back down, so we know that a shift isn't starting.

Then, on Day 16 she has a temp which looks a little elevated at 97.8. The next day is at 98.0 and the temps seem to go up from there. So by Day 19 she actually has four temperatures which look like a shift ... except for the fact that the one temp on Day 12 is really high and seems to be throwing things off.

What should she do?

PRACTICE CHART 3 : All Three Signs

In this case, she should discount that temp on Day 12.
Maybe she didn't sleep well or something else disturbed her temperature that night. Whatever the culprit, it is possible to disregard one of the temperatures in the six days before a shift if it seems to be an outlier compared to the others. Having five days of reliable data still gives you enough information.

So she would discount Day 12 and then set her Coverline based on the highest of the remaining temperatures. The highest value was 97.7, so the Coverline goes at 97.8.

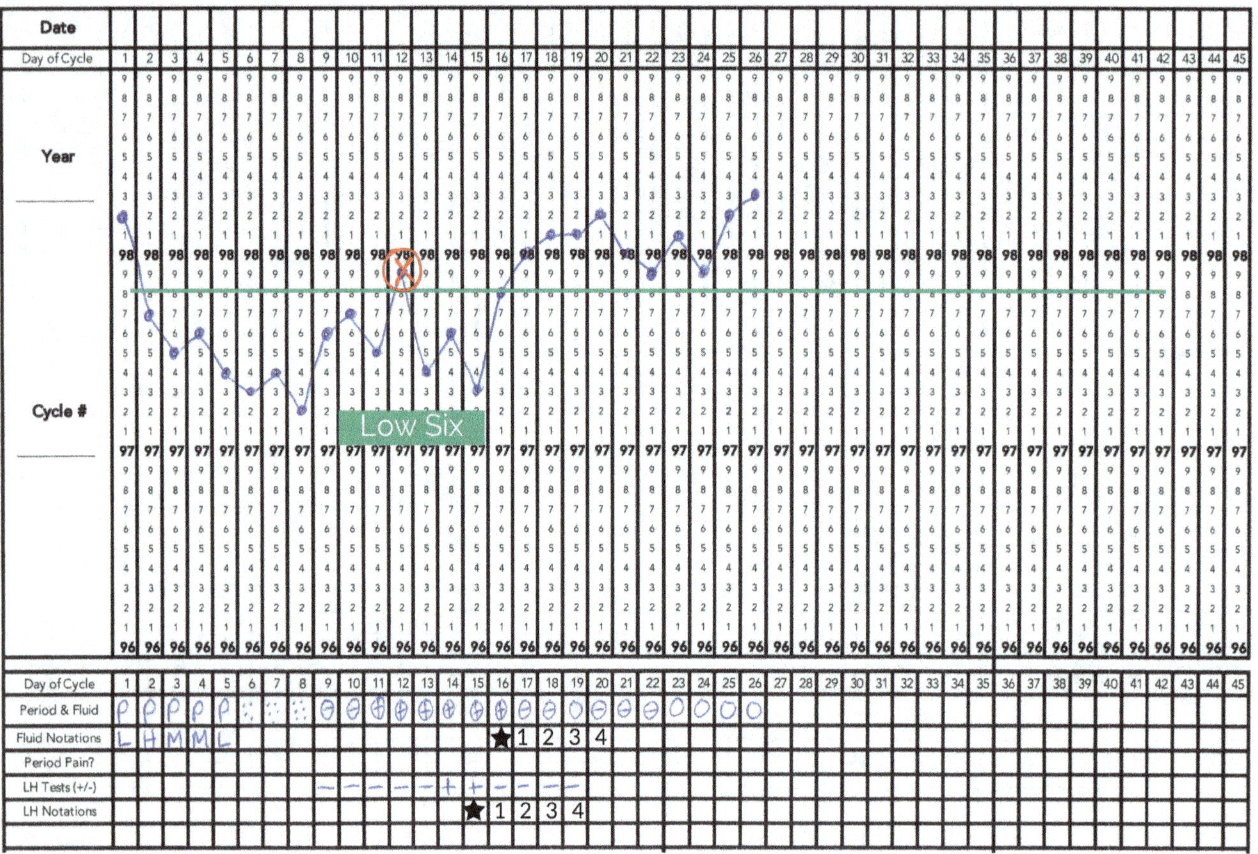

But now look what happens! She has a temperature sitting right on the Coverline. Day 16 is one of the temperatures she used to help identify the set of low six, but it's not high *enough* to count as the start of her shift.

When this happens, you can just skip over that day and begin counting with the next day, when the temp is very clearly above the Coverline.

Day 17 becomes the official start of the shift so she has four high temperatures by Day 20, which matches the count after Fluid Peak. LH count was met by Day 19, so **all three signs agree that ovulation has passed by Day 20.**

PRACTICE CHART 4: Fluid and LH Tests

For our next example, let's consider a woman who prefers to just use fluid and LH tests on her chart. This is an excellent option if you have irregular sleep schedules and don't want to invest in a more expensive temperature-tracking device.

In this example, she begins collecting LH Test data on Day 12. Perhaps she knows that she tends to have longer cycles and she doesn't want to use as many test sticks.

Date																							
Day of Cycle	1	2	3	4	5	6	7	8	9	10	11	12	13	14	15	16	17	18	19	20	21	22	23
Period & Fluid	P	P	P	P	P	P	O	⊖	⊖	⊖	⊖	⊖	⊖	⊕	⊕	⊖	⊕	⊕	⊕	⊖	⊖	⊖	⊖
Fluid Notations	L	M	L	L	L	L													★	1	2	3	4
Period Pain?																							
LH Tests (+/-)												−	−	−	−	−	−	−	−	+	−	−	−
LH Notations																				★	1	2	3

Date																						
Day of Cycle	24	25	26	27	28	29	30	31	32	33	34	35	36	37	38	39	40	41	42	43	44	45
Period & Fluid	O	O	O	O	O	O	O	O														
Fluid Notations																						
Period Pain?																						
LH Tests (+/-)	−																					
LH Notations	4																					

This combination of signs is perhaps the easiest to calculate, because you're simply looking for Fluid Peak Day and LH Peak Day.

Note that in this example, she starts to see Peak Type fluid on Day 14 and 15. The fluid switches to Non-Peak on Day 16, but then the Peak Type reappears on Day 17 and continues through Day 19. This means that Fluid Peak Day is Day 19 and the count after peak is complete by Day 23 with that sign.

She only got one positive (+) LH Test, which appeared on Day 20. That would be her LH Peak Day, which means that her count after LH peak is satisfied by Day 24.

Both signs agree that ovulation has likely passed by Day 24.

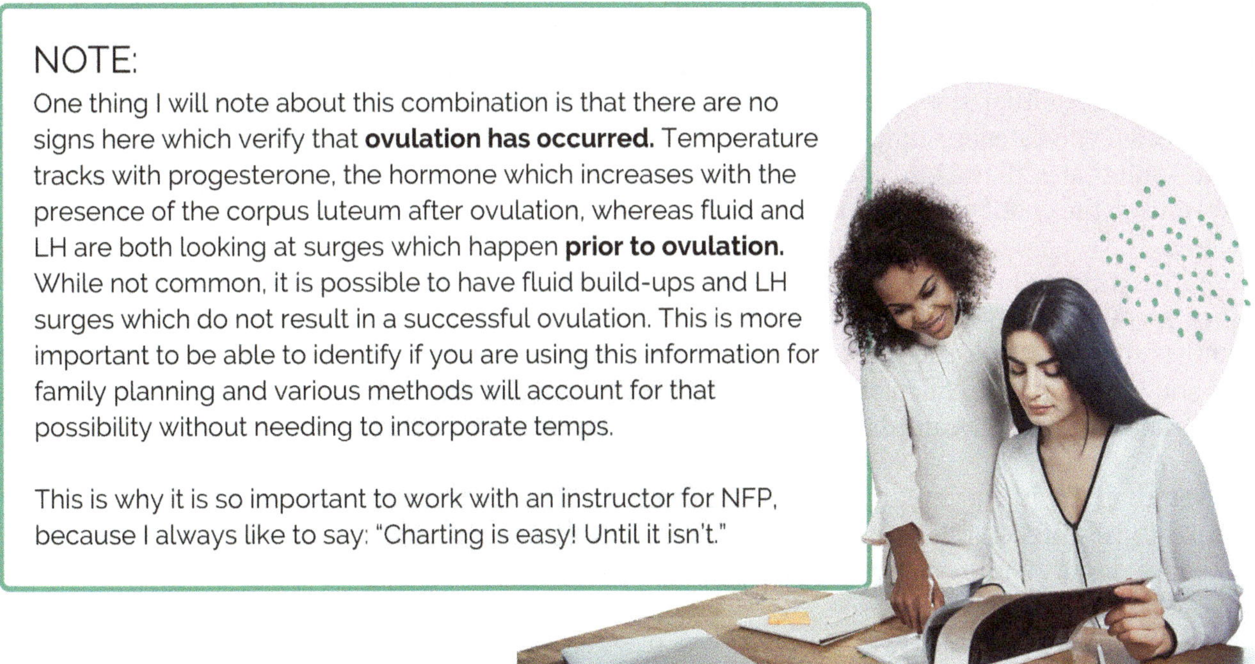

NOTE:

One thing I will note about this combination is that there are no signs here which verify that **ovulation has occurred.** Temperature tracks with progesterone, the hormone which increases with the presence of the corpus luteum after ovulation, whereas fluid and LH are both looking at surges which happen **prior to ovulation.** While not common, it is possible to have fluid build-ups and LH surges which do not result in a successful ovulation. This is more important to be able to identify if you are using this information for family planning and various methods will account for that possibility without needing to incorporate temps.

This is why it is so important to work with an instructor for NFP, because I always like to say: "Charting is easy! Until it isn't."

PRACTICE CHART 5: Fluid and BBT

Charting fluid and temps together is commonly referred to as a "sympto-thermal" approach. "Sympto" comes from the fluid sign, and "thermal" comes from the temperature sign. In order to verify ovulation with this chart, we find both Fluid Peak Day and a Temp Shift.

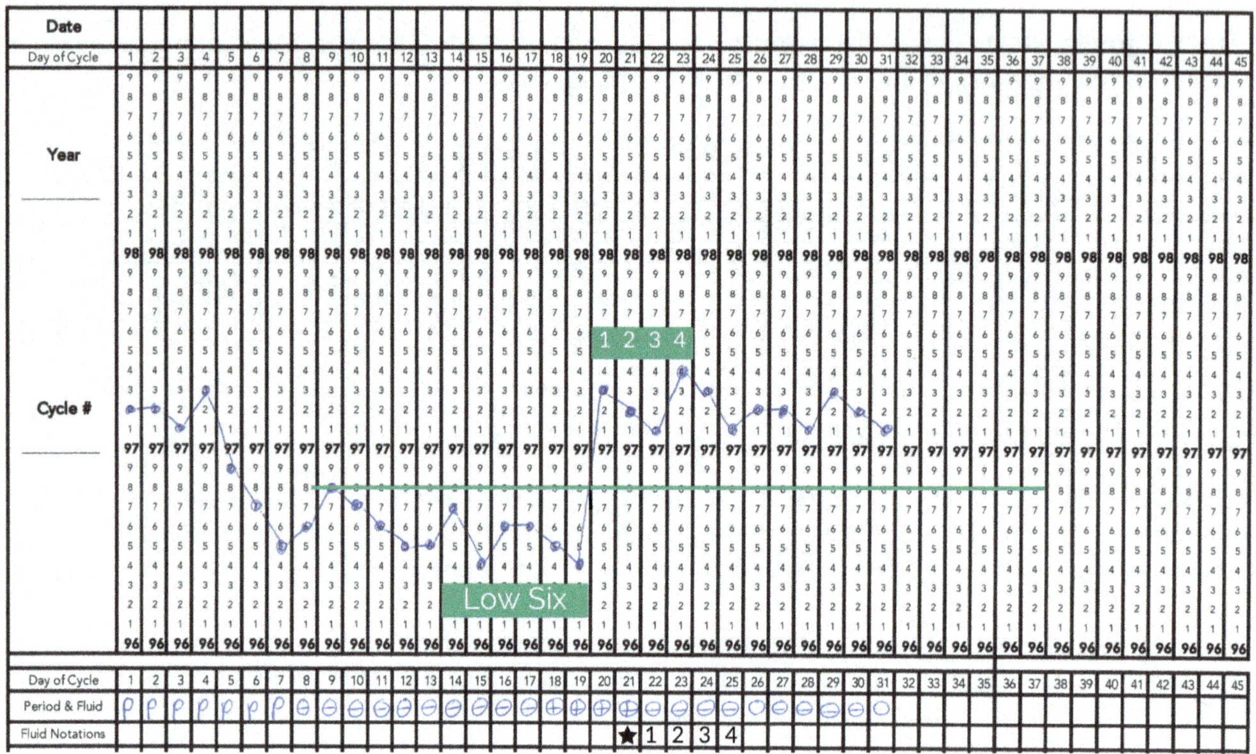

There are a couple of interesting things I wanted to show on this chart:
Starting with the fluid sign, notice that this woman has only recorded two Dry category days throughout the whole cycle. A lot of women worry that having constant fluid signs will mean that you can't accurately chart, but notice that it doesn't really matter if she has fluid all the time: what really matters is that she is able to tell the difference between her Non-Peak category fluid and hear Peak Type category fluid. Looking at this chart, she clearly marked four days of Peak Type fluid—and that's all the info she needed! The last day of Peak Type fluid was on Day 21 (Fluid Peak Day) and so the count after fluid peak is completed by Day 25.

The other thing to note is the range of her temperatures, which sit significantly lower than the other practice charts we have looked at. Some women typically see temps in this lower range, whether that's because their BBT is actually lower or because their device is calibrated lower. What this shows is that temp calculations are truly *relative*, so whether your temps tend to be high or low on the chart itself, all we need to verify is a shift with the range YOU experience.

We see that she has a very clear shift starting on Day 20 with a Coverline at 96.8, meaning her temperature shift count is satisfied by Day 23. This is a couple of days ahead of the fluid sign, so she would need to wait until Day 25 for both signs to agree that ovulation has passed.

Also note on this chart that she has a few days of temps which still look "high" at the beginning of her cycle. Some women will not notice a drop in temperatures until a few days into their bleed, but most women tend to see a drop right around Cycle Day 1.

PRACTICE CHART 6: BBT and LH Tests

Our final combination of signs is temperatures with LH tests. This is a great option for women who feel like they have scant fluid signs or who simply don't want to observe a single sign throughout the day. The temperature data is taken first thing in the morning, and LH tests are done just once per day, so they require less attention on a regular basis. For this combination, we will need to identify a Temp Shift and LH Peak Day.

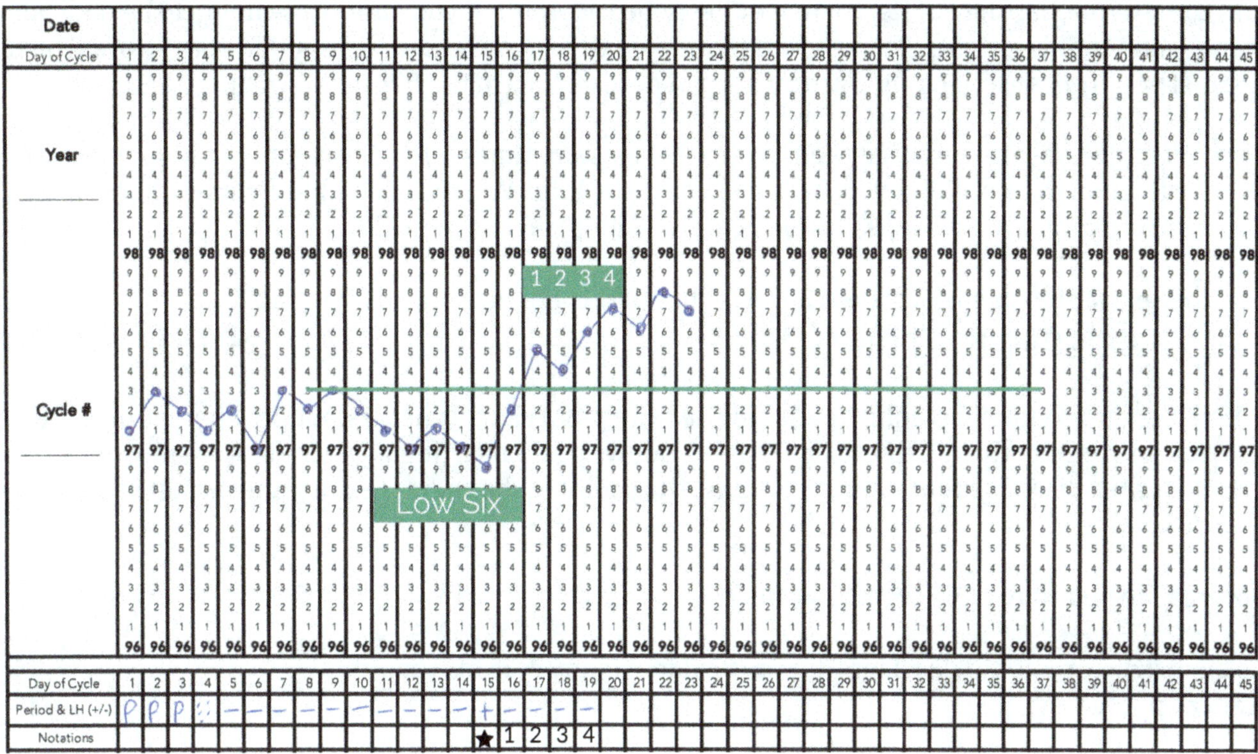

Note that in this chart, she only has one day where she gets a positive (+) LH test. That will automatically be her LH Peak Day, which means that her count after LH Peak is satisfied by Day 19.

The temperature calculation is fairly straightforward as well. On Day 17 she sees a temperature higher than the six before it, which is followed by three more days of elevated temps. Her Coverline gets set at 97.3 because the highest value in the Low Six was 97.2. She then counts four temperatures above the line and satisfies the Temp Shift count by Day 20.

Thus, both LH and temperature agree that ovulation has passed by Day 20.

Letting Go of "Perfect"

Notice that on every single practice chart I just showed you, all of the women were charting all of their chosen data every day. They could identify ovulation with each sign and things lined up fairly well each time.

I want to conclude this section by reminding you that even if you manage to develop very strong and consistent charting habits, there will likely be times when you simply cannot get the data you want— and that is alright! Sickness, travel, broken thermometers, or stressful days at work which distract you from observing fluid are all normal occurrences in the lives of women.

Even more normal are signs that seem not to line up sometimes, or temperature readings which are just "off" enough to prohibit you from calculating a shift. You may even have a medical condition which directly impacts the appearance of certain data points on your chart.

One thing I want to emphasize here is that your chart is not meant to be "perfect."
Your chart is meant to be useful.

When it comes to family planning, a lot of the utility of a chart is dependent on whether or not the couple can confidently identify their fertile window. When charting as a single woman who is not yet concerned directly about family planning, the utility of the chart is pretty much what you decide it to be.

So, what do you want to use your chart for?

As an instructor, my single clients have articulated many reasons that they want to pursue charting:

> *"I want to see if my migraines are actually lining up with my hormonal shifts. How my doctor will treat my headaches is somewhat dependent on whether they have a hormonal component."*
>
> *"I am worried about infertility, since I know my mom had trouble conceiving. I'm not engaged yet, but think it would be good to know if my charts show any signs of problems —because then I can invest in working with a doctor before I actually try to start a family."*
>
> *"I've been working with a holistic doctor who is helping me with changes in my diet, but she didn't really know how to help me track my cycles to see if that is impacting my other symptoms. Would you be able to help me chart these things to see how they correlate with ovulation?"*
>
> *"I've suffered from really awful PMS my entire life. I think if I had a better sense of when mood changes might be coming, I could prepare better. And I would also know why these things are happening. I don't want to blame my cycle. But if I'm having a hard time, it's also nice to know there could be a reason, and that some of my moods will resolve once my period starts."*

Letting Go of "Perfect"

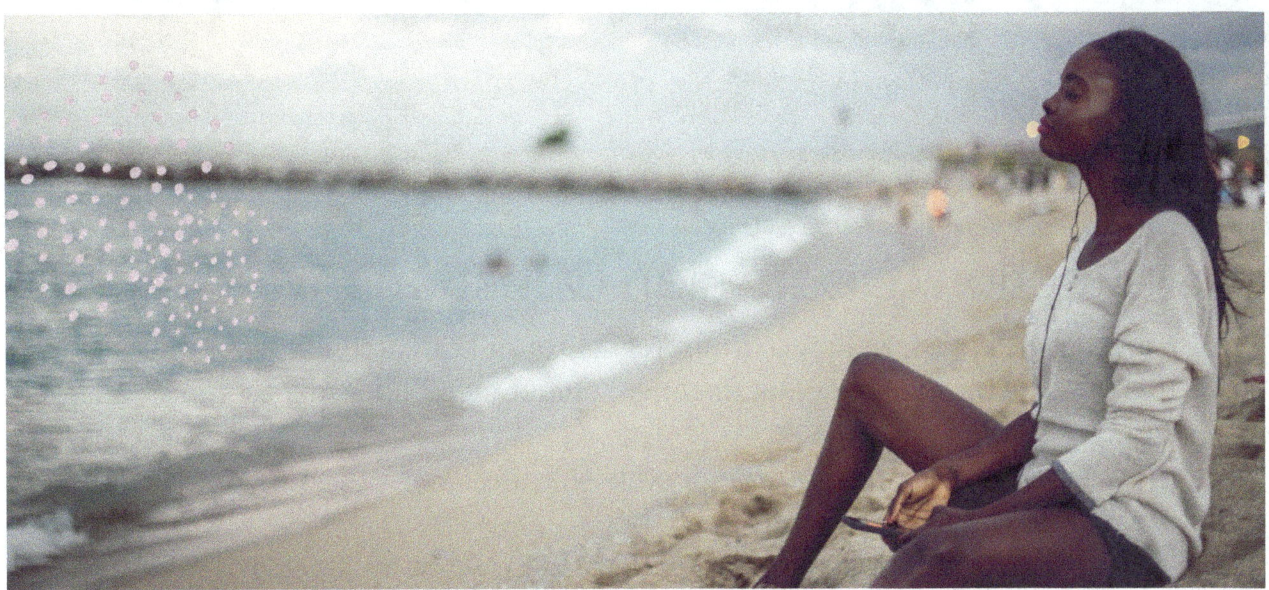

It's good to get in the habit of doing a little "check in" with yourself once in a while, and to invite God into the conversation about how charting may be positively or negatively impacting your life at the moment. What are you gaining? What is challenging? Is charting creating any new issues or raising new questions for you?

In my field, it's very common for instructors to suggest that *every woman needs to chart!* But cycle charting requires consistency, commitment, and a firm sense of motivation. If there is no *need* for you to chart, then you shouldn't put undue pressure on yourself to do so.

Ideally, charting your cycle would be a positive experience of gaining self-knowledge: **our Faith tells us that knowledge is intimately tied to love, so knowledge about myself should be a source of love and respect for myself as a creature, as a woman with her own unique dignity and worth.** And acknowledging the Goodness in myself should also be a source of knowledge about the Creator which leads to deeper love of God and neighbor.

So another motivation, which takes charting to another deeper level is to say:

"As a single woman, I'd like to grow more comfortable in my female body. I think that will help me in my relationship with God, because I struggle to see the Goodness of my body sometimes."

For many women—actually, I think for most women—this "ideal" is obscured by the reality of painful periods, shame, embarrassment, or just a lack of comfort and familiarity with our bodies. It's not all sunshine and roses when it comes to charting our cycles! Learning to read the *Language of the Body* in this very particular way is a skill which can take a long time to become comfortable with. But of course we have a loving God who knows all of this and is unceasingly patient with us.

As you begin your practice of charting, it is my prayer that you can extend that same patience to yourself! Let go of "perfect" and give yourself permission to chart (or not chart!) your cycles according to your own goals and preferences.

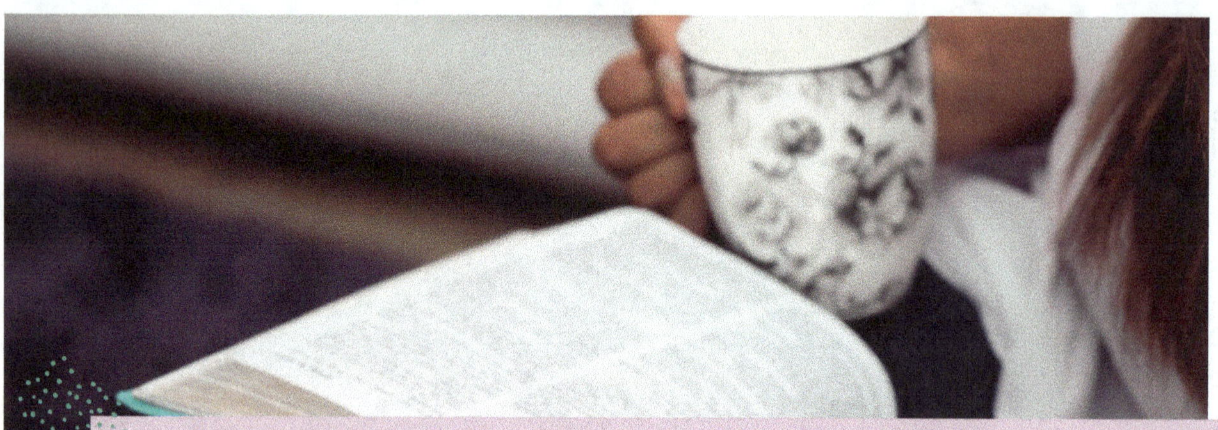

Reflection/Discussion Questions

Now that we have seen how to interpret charts and can better understand what this practice may look like, let us reflect on our own hopes, expectations, and fears:

- What do I hope to gain through cycle charting? What is going to make my chart feel useful in my daily life?
- Do I have a hard time letting go of perfection? What might God be asking of me as I take up this practice of cycle charting?
- Do I have any fears or concerns about the knowledge I may gain through cycle charting? How can I invite God to walk with me through this experience? Is there anyone else I can think of who could walk with me?
- I am only just now uncovering this information about myself, but God has known it from the moment of my existence. God designed and intimately knows my unique cycle. How does this make me feel?

"It is ridiculous to think that we can enter Paradise without first entering ourselves! We must get to know ourselves, reflect on our limitations, acknowledge our gratitude for God, and solicit his mercy."
–St. Teresa of Avila

"Before I formed you in the womb, I knew you, and before you were born I consecrated you."
–Jeremiah 1:5

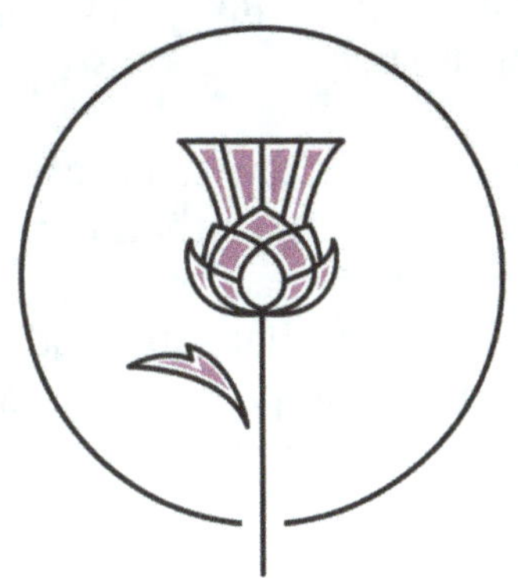

INTEGRATING
CHARTING INTO MY LIFE

Charting at the Service of Holiness

Now that you've learned how to keep a chart and have an idea of the valuable information this practice may contain, it's worth pausing to reflect a little further on how charting integrates into our lives. I hesitate to say that cycle charting is a *lifestyle,* though many people have referred to the use of NFP and the practice of charting as such.

That term does capture the fact that learning how to observe, chart, and interpret our biological cycle signs is something that impacts much more than our bathroom routines. Much like other *lifestyle* modifications, it has the potential to impact our entire mindset about what it means to live in this body and to pursue certain goals within that same body. For example, choosing to switch to a heathy diet is a lifestyle choice. It not only impacts the food which goes into our mouths, but it will impact our shopping choices, where we spend our social time, and how we think about other things we put into our bodies besides food. So in that sense, perhaps charting is like a *lifestyle* choice.

On the other hand, charting should not be something around which our entire life revolves. It should not constitute a *lifestyle* in and of itself because **as Christians, the pursuit of holiness should actually be our lifestyle**. So, anything we do—including our attempts to monitor biological health —should be seen as actions at the service of holiness, and as integrated parts of our efforts to get ourselves and our loved ones to heaven.

How can we do that?
I think Pope St. John Paul II offers us some good food for thought when he discusses pregnancy in *Mulieris dignitatem:*

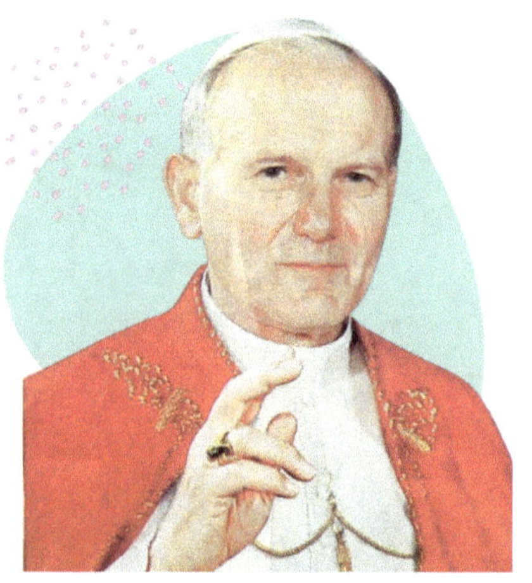

> What the different branches of science have to say on this subject is important and useful, provided that it is not limited to an exclusively bio-physiological interpretation of women and of motherhood. Such a "restricted" picture would go hand in hand with a materialistic concept of the human being and of the world. In such a case, **what is truly essential would unfortunately be lost.**

In other words, we must not allow our practice of cycle charting to narrow our self-focus and reflection down to our purely materialistic (bodily) existence. Hopefully you have noticed that our reflection questions so far have tried to link charting with contemplation of God, self, and spiritual discipline. It is of fundamental importance that we, as women, understand how our bodies are integral to our identity as beloved daughters of God. They are not inconsequential as we seek holiness!

However, in trying to rightfully understand for ourselves what God has pronounced good, we must not over-emphasize our bodies to the detriment of the spirit. We must remember the truly essential reality: that we are both body and soul, together.

Charting at the Service of Holiness

Ok, Christina, that's some good talk right there. But practically speaking, what does that mean?

A very wise professor once told me: "Nobody speaks from nowhere." What he meant was that we bring our unique experiences, situations, gifts, and challenges to every conversation. This holds true even when we think about the conversation our bodies speak to and about God: when it comes to understanding and integrating the *Language of the Body* into our daily lives, nobody speaks from nowhere.

So, precisely how you keep focus on your whole self is going to be determined largely by your own unique experiences, thoughts, and challenges. If you are someone who has struggled with body image, for example, you will need to integrate charting into your broader efforts to heal from that struggle. I do not think it would therefore be helpful for me to enumerate a list of specific ways in which women dealing with specific struggles *should* approach their process of embracing and integrating cycle awareness into their experience of self. But I will offer some general advice about what I think is required for us to honor what is truly essential:

- *Bring your bodily needs, concerns, and joys with you when you approach God in prayer. Do not consider them less worthy of His attention than your spiritual needs.*
- *Dive deeply into the rich graces offered through the Sacraments, which show for us exactly how our bodies are meant to be physical receptacles and vehicles of God's presence in the world.*
- *Engage your body in prayer. Pay close attention to the ways in which we pray with our bodies during Mass, and consider utilizing those gestures in your devotional prayer as well. An easy way to start is by bowing your head at the name of Jesus, or when praying a doxology.*
- *Stay close to the saints, especially female saints and, of course, our Blessed Mother. Ask them to pray for you and invite them to instruct you in what they have learned about their identity as unique and unrepeatable images of God.*
- *Be honest with yourself about whether charting is harming your sense of self-worth, or your relationships with God and others. If so, try to discern whether this interference may be a form of spiritual attack, designed to keep you from embracing the goodness of your body. Give yourself permission to stop charting while you figuring things out, and to pick it up again when you are ready.*

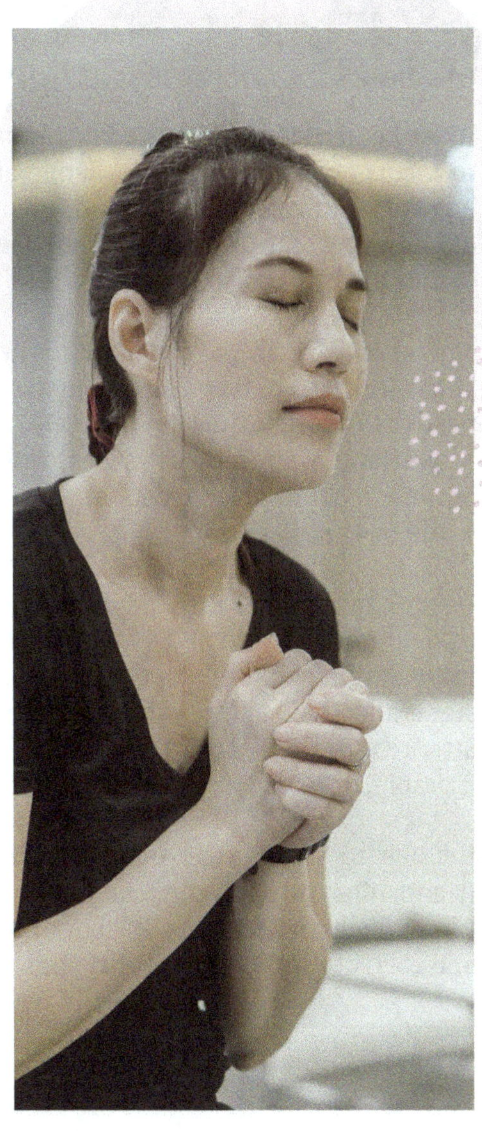

The Adjustment Period

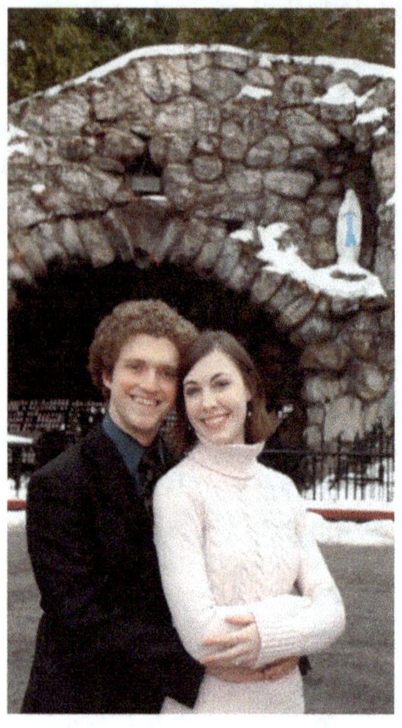

I first started charting my cycle when I was engaged, because I hadn't thought to start charting before that time. What I experienced in those few months before the wedding was, honestly, a little bit disorienting. I would wake up, take my temperature, and think to myself, "Ah, I am probably fertile today." But having that be one of my first thoughts of the day—as a woman who was not yet ready to act on that information—felt incongruous. As I tried to remain chaste in thought and action with my fiancé, I didn't like the daily reminder which turned my thoughts to sex and babies.

As I learned more about my cycles, I also realized that I was also starting to analyze my moods and behaviors in the context of cycle phases. *Why am I feeling irritable today? Is it just because I'm in my luteal phase?* It felt a little bit like I had lost a sense of autonomy, as I became aware of the ways my hormones impacted my reactions to various situations and people. Was I just being controlled by hormones?

What I experienced in those few months was merely an adjustment time, a time when I was trying to incorporate this new knowledge about my body not only into all of the other things I already knew about myself, but also into my relationships and interactions with other people. It was a sort of paradigm shift, which made me feel disoriented and little bit awkward while I was transitioning through it.

Now that I am on the other side, I no longer worry about any lack of agency when I notice mood shifts. On the contrary, I actually have a better sense of my personal strengths, weaknesses, and needs at different times in my cycle, and I make a conscious effort to be proactive about addressing or working around those issues, rather than always being reactive in the moment. Charting has become a habit which exists in the background of my life, rather than taking a front seat as it did while I was still learning.

Despite my early challenges, it has become something that is just a natural part of life—something I do so my husband and I can plan our family, but also something I do which gives me valuable information about my health and state of mind. Learning how to pay attention to my own body's signs and the way my moods and energy levels shift through my cycle has also made me more attentive to the needs of other women. It helps me to be more magnanimous if my friend seems irritable, or to be more respectful when someone tries to draw boundaries for social time.

I'd like to share a story to illustrate the particular point that cycle awareness can help our friendships, through the lens of one of my young Cycle Prep participants. Cycle Prep is a course I offer which teaches girls all about cycles, periods, and how to create a *Culture of Care* for ourselves and each other throughout the whole cycle. Here is what one mother shared:

The Adjustment Period

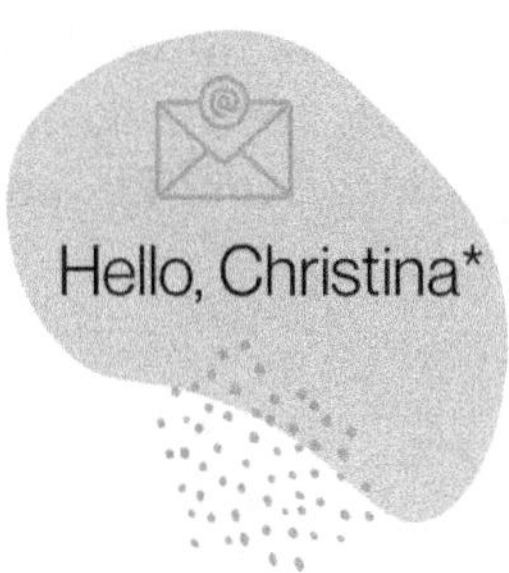

My daughter and I did your Cycle Prep course, and a few days after that she was expecting to go on a hiking trip with one of her best friends. They had been planning this for a long time, but the morning of the hike, her friend called and said she didn't feel up to hiking. She canceled and I just knew that my daughter was crushed. Before Cycle Prep, she probably would have gotten really angry at this friend and been in quite the mood all day. But instead she said something which surprised me: "Mom, I wonder if my friend is on her period or maybe in her luteal phase. Maybe her body is telling her that she needs to rest instead of going on this hike. I'd still like to hang out with her. Do you think we could call her back and invite her to watch a movie instead?"

Sure enough, we called back and the friend was happy to switch plans. The girls had a great time, all because my daughter was aware enough to think that something was going on physically, rather than assuming that the girl just didn't want to spend time with her.

I love this story because it shows how small, simple acts of respecting our body signals can lead to decreased "drama" in relationships and new opportunities to share time together!

Cycles do not need to be the lens through which we see all of our interactions, but they can be one more way we seek to understand, respect, and love each other as sisters in Christ. And charting allows my husband to better understand me, as well!

Finding out all of this new information about ourselves can be empowering, but it can also feel overwhelming. This is why I believe so firmly that single women should be invited to learn how to chart, because body literacy is like any other form of literacy: **it takes time to become fluent.**

Think about it this way: learning to "read" our cycle is like learning how to read Shakespeare.
When we teach our children how to read, do we begin with Shakespeare? *No!* They first need to learn the alphabet and which letters make certain sounds, then they learn about sound combinations and how to form simple words ... and so on until they are finally ready.

In other words, we understand that building literacy takes time and you simply cannot do it all at once. We also know that literacy is different from fluency. We should expect that incorporating cycle charting into your life will take some time and require some adjustments. You may be someone who wants to start with charting and then proceed to deeper reflection once you've got the mechanics down. Or perhaps you are someone who prefers to contemplate the deeper meaning of our bodies *before* you enter into charting. Likely, it will be an ever deepening and expanding experience of both those things simultaneously.

I believe this sort of learning is consonant with our Catholic Faith. After all, our God did not reveal Himself in one instant, but unfolded His self-revelation over thousands of years. So give yourself permission to take it slowly and to gradually grow in these habits as you dive into this aspect of the *mystery* of your womanhood.

**slightly paraphrased from conversation*

Talking About Charting

When we think about integrating charting into our lives, a few questions may arise about whether or how to talk to others about this practice. Do we need to tell everyone about it? Should we keep it to ourselves? I hope by now that you can anticipate my answer to be: "That depends a lot on *you!*"

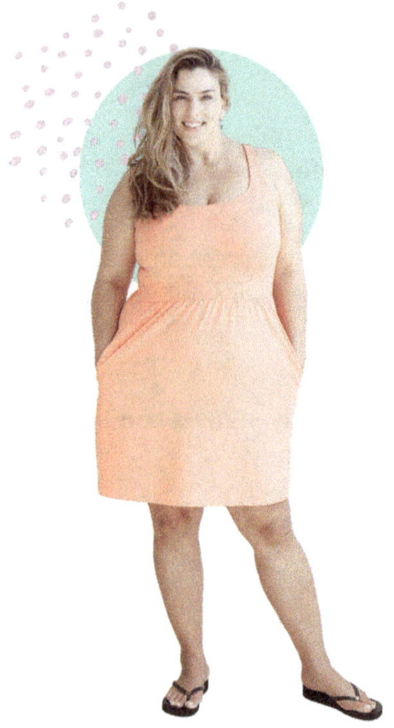

FOR THE WOMAN WHO JUST LOVES TO TALK ABOUT IT

Some women love the process of cycle charting so much that they cannot help but interject it into conversations with friends, family, and even the occasional stranger. If this is your gift, I do not think you need to shy away from it; however, your challenge will be to consider the receptivity of others to hearing this message. It may be the case that your friend who is looking to ditch hormonal birth control is looking for precisely this answer! But it may also be the case that, for any number of reasons, this suggestion feels scary, intimidating, or downright stupid. I won't lie: some people have serious misconceptions that cycle charting is completely "woo" and not based on science. In that case, gentle invitations and a slower introduction to the idea of charting, coupled with the promise that you will accompany her, are going to be more productive. Don't give up on sharing this practice with your friends if they are not receptive at the first mention! But also don't be so enthused about telling everyone that you forget to take their situation and feelings into account.

FOR THE WOMAN WHO DOESN'T WANT TO TALK ABOUT IT

If you are more comfortable not talking about cycle charting, then feel free to keep this to yourself. As long as there is no one who is directly impacted by your charting (like, a future spouse or a doctor) that you need to talk to, it's perfectly fine to have this be a private part of your life that you do not share with others; but be aware that there's a difference between holding something reverently as a private and personal experience, and hiding it because you're ashamed or embarrassed. It is the hope that your experience would be the former, rather than the latter.

Keep in mind, however, that there may be times when people notice your charting and ask about it! If you have roommates, for example, it's possible they may see your LH tests in the trash (they look a lot like pregnancy tests), or you may have people ask you why you always set your alarm for the same time even when you don't plan to get up. In these cases, you could decline to answer, but I also think it is prudent to heed the advice of St. Peter: "Always be prepared to give an answer to everyone who asks you to give the reason for the hope that you have" (1 Peter 3:15). In other words, it can be an act of charity to share about the benefits you have gained from cycle charting when someone directly asks. You never know what a gift you may be giving that person through inviting them to know more about their body and their health.

Talking About Charting

FOR THE WOMAN WHO WANTS TO TALK TO A BOYFRIEND

If you have plans for using this information for Natural Family Planning in the future, it's important to talk about this with a potential spouse. Couples will have their own timelines for talking about questions of children and family life: some jump in fairly early, while others take longer. Whatever your timeline is, don't shy away from including the "how" question in discussions about family planning. Be prepared to discuss **why** NFP is important to you, and then you can share **what** you are already doing as an investment towards that future possibility. Be attentive to his response because a man who has never thought about using NFP may have one initial reaction and then come around to your point of view later. Men truly desire what is best for the health and wellbeing of the women they love, so they may actually be open to this new idea out of respect for you, even if they are not initially interested for themselves. If you do become engaged, be sure to invite him to attend NFP classes with you so the two of you can learn how to incorporate charting into your shared family planning experience.

TIPS FOR TALKING WITH A BOYFRIEND:

1. Be prudent about over-sharing. The details of your chart and the particular ways of observing biomarkers are not things that you need to cover in the beginning. Initial conversations should be about the *idea* of charting, rather than the specifics.
2. You don't have to be the expert: Don't feel that you need to explain everything to him yourself. Offer the information that you feel confident sharing, and then offer to read, watch, or study other resources together to answer more of his questions.
3. Focus on why this is important to you. Remember that your reasons matter!
4. Remember that men have likely been taught for their entire lives that using condoms or other forms of contraception was the responsible and loving thing to do. Help him to see the practicality of this other option by discussing the medical and health standpoint, the efficacy of different methods, and Church teaching which supports this as the option which preserves dignity and love for both spouses.
5. Make sure he knows that he would be included in NFP. Cycle charting may be a personal habit for you right now, but family planning is a shared responsibility that he would have a part in, too.

Talking About Charting

FOR THE WOMAN WHO NEEDS TO TALK WITH A DOCTOR

There are a few different reasons you might need (or want) to bring up charting with a doctor. You may need to show your chart to a provider in the context of a check-up, or to assist with investigation or diagnosis with some health issues. If you're preparing to talk to your doctor in one of these situations, keep in mind that not all doctors will be knowledgeable about modern NFP/FAM methods or necessarily supportive, but they are an important part of your care team regardless!

Doctors are perfectly capable of respecting your decision, even if they do not have personal experience with these methods. In general, a relationship with your doctor will be easy to maintain if your doctor:

- is not outright dismissive of your choice to use NFP.
- is comfortable discussing menstrual patterns or cycle concerns as part of regular care.
- is open to hearing your interpretation of charts, even if they cannot read the chart themselves.
- is willing to refer you to specialists to help with any cycle concerns.

If you are uncomfortable with your doctor's response, you can check out the *Resources* section for information on finding a provider.

Another reason you may need to talk about charting with your doctor is in the context of therapy. It is possible to use your charts to track hormonally-influenced symptoms like PMDD, anxiety, depression, or even ADHD.

Additionally, learning how to "read" our body and to work with it in this very intimate way can be hugely healing and therapeutic, or it can cause previous issues to resurface or manifest in different ways. Sometimes it can be a little bit of both. I have worked with women for whom charting is a path to healing from many types of trauma and shame, but I also have clients for whom this sort of intimacy with their bodies is a bit of an obstacle.

Remember in these cases that mental health is a part of your *whole self health* and being honest about the benefits or challenges of charting in these particular contexts can be part of constructive conversations with your doctor, and also with your self.

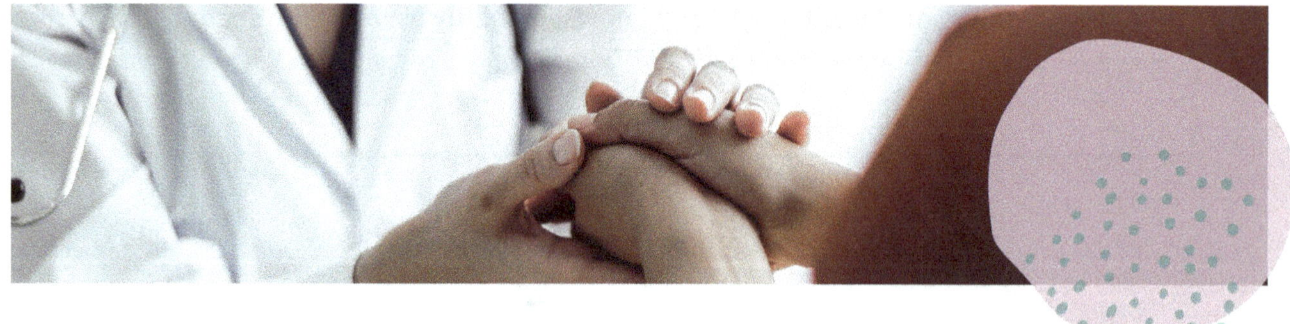

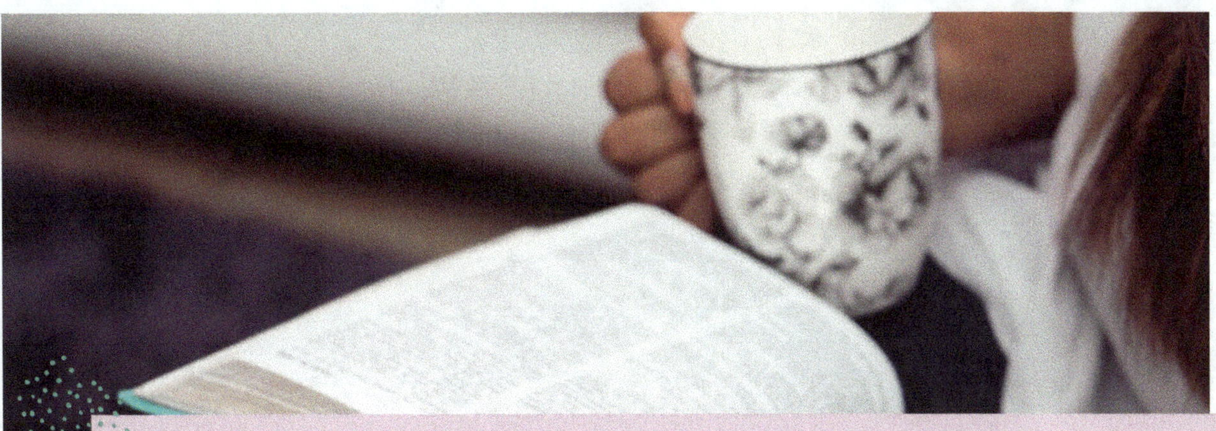

Reflection/Discussion Questions

As you think about integrating charting and cycle knowledge into your life, remember that changes may come gradually! Allow yourself to enter into this time of transition, reflecting on the following:

- How does learning this about my body, in my single state of life, challenge me to see the value of my body in and of itself (not just in relationship to men)?
- What questions do I still have about insights I could gain through charting? Does the thought of charting carry any concerns?
- If charting helps me discover more about my mood patterns, can I think of ways that might help me be more patient and gentle with myself?
- What difference might it make in my relationships and prayer life to know that my cycle may impact how I feel?

"The meaning of the specifically feminine being is not to be understood only by her relation to man... All creatures relate to God in their divine likeness; thus it is befitting the feminine nature that her characteristic function is to reflect the divine."
–St. Edith Stein

"I am created by God, and for this purpose alone: To praise and serve him, and so enter eternal life; and not only to praise and serve him in any state of life, but in this state in which he desires me, and to which he has called me."
–Ven. Bruno Lanteri, O.M.V.

Journal Page

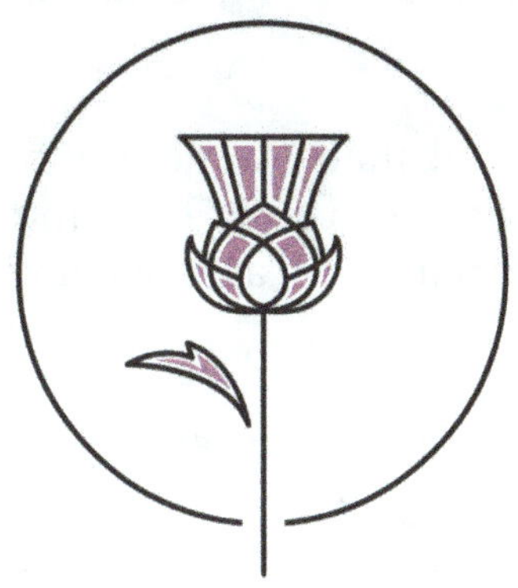

RESOURCES

Different Methods of NFP

If you're ready to start learning a method for family planning, use the following resources to find one that works for you! **This list is neither exhaustive nor authoritative regarding USCCB-approved methods of NFP. All sites listed according to information available as of October 2022.**

OVULATION METHODS
Use a single fertility indicator—cervical fluid—to determine the fertile window for the couple. These methods require no extra devices, generally have minimal ongoing costs, and tend to be great for couples who are confident working with a lot of detail on a single sign.

- Billings USA: boma-usa.org
- Creighton Model: creightonmodel.com, naprotechnology.com, fertilitycare.org
- Family of the Americas: familyplanning.net
- FEMM (with optional sympto-hormonal): femmhealth.org

SYMPTO-THERMAL METHODS
Use two indicators—cervical fluid and temperature—to determine the fertile window for the couple. Traditional temperatures can be difficult for shift-workers, parents of small children, or anyone with irregular sleep patterns and may require investment in a specialized thermometer for best efficacy. Couples may appreciate that these methods offer confirmation of fertility from multiple signs.

- Couple to Couple League: ccli.org
- NFP International: nfpandmore.org
- Sensiplan: replyobgyn.com/services/sensiplan/
- SymptoPro: symptopro.org

HORMONAL METHODS (sometimes referred to as "sympto-hormonal")
May use a variety of indicators to determine fertility, but always have hormone monitoring as their distinctive feature. These methods are the most rapidly-evolving category and generally require the highest level of financial investments, both upfront and ongoing. Couples may appreciate the objectivity and confidence which comes from hormone measurements, especially when paired with other fertility indicators to confirm ovulation.

- Boston Cross Check: bostoncrosscheck.com
- Marquette Model: marquette.edu/nursing/natural-family-planning.php
- FEMM: femmhealth.org

CALENDAR-BASED METHODS
Although they tend to get bad press (and most physicians assume all "NFP" is the same as the "rhythm method"), the classic rhythm method and its more modern cousins can be very simple means of NFP if a client meets certain cycle criteria for regularity and length. Couples should work with a trained instructor to assess whether they meet that criteria.

- CycleBeads: cyclebeads.com
- Standard Days Method (General info): irh.org/standard-days-method

Other Tracking Devices

This guide has presented you with three primary options for charting biomarkers, but the world of femtech and biodata monitoring is constantly evolving! In addition to the devices and techniques already listed here, you may want to investigate:

Clearblue Fertility Monitor

This hormone monitoring device measures LH, but also looks at estrogen (in the form of estradiol). It assesses these two hormones based on preset thresholds, but also by baseline measurements for the individual woman. Results will show low, high, and peak to determine a fertile window leading up to ovulation. This device is not designed specifically for postponing pregnancy, but is an approved device for both Boston Cross Check and Marquette for NFP. Protocols for using this device for NFP should be learned from a trained provider.

Tempdrop

This wearable thermometer uses axillary temperature measurements, taken throughout the night, to determine a woman's basal body temperature. It does not have independent efficacy studies which prove that its measurements can be utilized in the same way oral/vaginal BBT can be used for NFP, but many methods have instructors who have worked with the device and will support users who wish to utilize it for charting. It can be a great option for anyone with irregular sleep schedules.

Proov

This at-home hormone monitoring company pioneered the PdG (progesterone) test, and continues to innovate by expanding their testing line to include LH tests and FSH (ovarian reserve) tests. Some methods offer instruction with these tests to confirm ovulation.

As of October 2022, the following devices represent **a small handful** of products which are also advertised for family planning use:

- Ava: wearable fertility tracker bracelet
- Cycle Beads: a modern approach to calendar-based tracking
- Daysy: fertility tracker and smart thermometer
- Kegg: cervical fluid tracker
- Lady Comp: digital thermometer and fertility tracker
- Mira: fertility monitor
- Natural Cycles: app-based family planning method
- Oova: combined LH and progesterone test
- Oura Ring: temperature tracking for cycle monitoring
- OvaCue: tracks electrolytes in saliva and cervical fluid
- OvuSense: vaginal temperature tracking and app

As interest in cycle charting grows, we should expect to see more devices come on the market. The important thing is to make sure that, prior to investing in any additional technology or devices, you consult with your chosen instructor about the suitability for that particular device with your method. Most femtech devices are currently produced for women who are trying to conceive, and the fertility market in the US alone is about $8 billion per year. You can imagine that not every one of the companies entering that market will be invested in producing materials suitable for Catholic use of NFP.

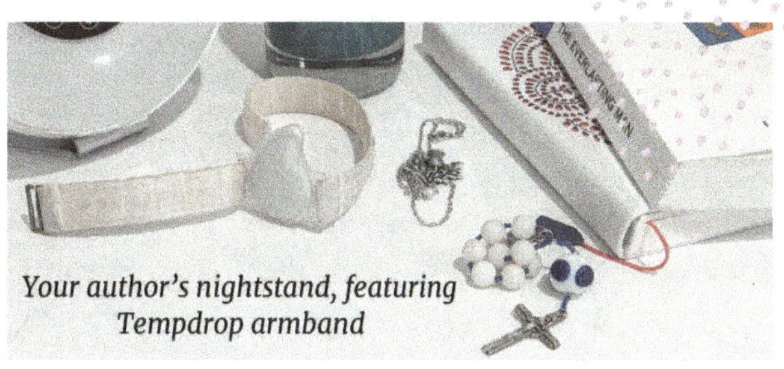

Your author's nightstand, featuring Tempdrop armband

Connecting With a Doctor

If your current doctor doesn't respond to your cycle charting in a way that you are comfortable with, here are some other resources and options you can consider:

- **Find a new doctor:** If you have options for another provider and you already know what you want to look for, don't be afraid to ask around. Your provider does not need to be able to teach NFP or work directly with a chart, but should respect your choice of family planning method.
- **Seek out additional help of someone who takes a "restorative reproductive medicine" approach:** This is a good option if you want to keep your doctor, but really want some assistance going deeper with integrating your cycles into your personal health. Providers taking this approach can be doctors or nurses, and may be found through NaProTECHNOLOGY Centers, FEMM Health, Billings Ovulation Method Association (BOMA), or the Marquette Model. Here are a few links to help you get connected with restorative reproductive medicine (RRM) providers and services:

My Catholic Doctor: offers pro-life telehealth services across the United States that include virtual visits, lab or imaging orders, and prescription requests.
mycatholicdoctor.com/our-services/family-planning

St. Paul VI Institute: National Hormone Lab, the hub for NaProTECHNOLOGY™ in the USA, can provide hormonal screening even with samples collected across state lines.
popepaulvi.com/laboratory

FEMM Medical Provider Directory:
femmhealth.org/medical-providers

Natural Womanhood: provides a list of doctors spanning various specialities who are committed to offering better care alternatives than hormonal contraceptives.
naturalwomanhood.org/about/doctors

Fertility Science Institute Directory: find a medical professional trained specifically within an FABM (NFP) system, or locate doctors who, despite not being trained in an FABM, are supportive of charting and allied to the principles of RRM.
fertilityscienceinstitute.org/directory/

Billings Medical Provider Directory:
boma-usa.org/billings-trained-physicians.html

A (Very Brief) List of Books

About Fertility Awareness/NFP and Women's Health

Please note: some of these books present barrier/backup options not in line with Church teaching.
If you are looking for scientific references for the materials covered in this text, this list is a GREAT place to start!

The Fifth Vital Sign- by Lisa Hendrickson-Jack
The Period Repair Manual- by Dr Lara Briden
Fertility, Cycles, and Nutrition- by Marilyn M. Shannon
Hormone Intelligence- by Dr Aviva Romm
The Complete Guide to Fertility Awareness- by Jane Knight
Taking Charge of Your Fertility- by Toni Weschler
Natural Family Planning: A Catholic Approach- by Mary Lee Barron
The Happy Girl's Guide to Being Whole- by Teresa Kenney

About Church Teaching and Theology of the Body

Casti connubii- by Pius XI
Humanae vitae- by Paul VI
Familiaris consortio- by John Paul II
Good News About Sex & Marriage- by Christopher West
Man and Woman He Created Them, a Theology of the Body- by John Paul II
Theology of the Body for Beginners- by Christopher West
Men and Women Are From Eden: A Study Guide to JP II's Theology of the Body- by Mary Healy
These Beautiful Bones: An Everyday Theology of the Body- by Emily Stimpson Chapman
The Genesis of Gender- by Abigail Favale

About Catholic Femininity

Mulieris dignitatem- by John Paul II
The Collected Works of Edith Stein- Volume Two: Essays on Women
Reveal the Gift: Living the Feminine Genius- by Lisa Cotter
Undone- by Carrie Schuchts Daunt
You Are Enough- by Danielle Bean
Letters to Women: Embracing the Feminine Genius in Everyday Life- by Chloe Langr
With All Her Mind: A Call to the Intellectual Life- ed. by Rachel Bulman

Other

The following books are not specifically Catholic resources, but touch on issues related to cycles and femininity.

Wholistic Feminism- by Leah A. Jacobson
A Brief Theology of Periods (Yes, Really!)- by Rachel Jones
Breaking Free From Body Shame: Dare to Reclaim what God Has Named Good- by Jess Connolly

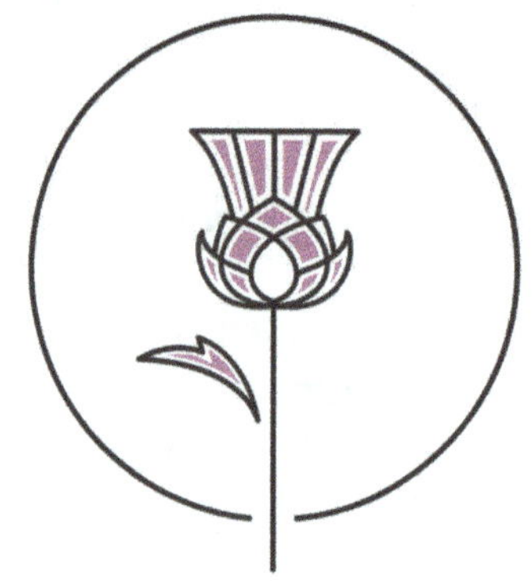

CHARTS

The following pages contain charts that you should feel free to copy and use directly if you'd like to keep a paper chart. Options given are:

- All three signs (BBT + FLUID + LH tests)
- Just Fluid + LH

If you are tracking temperatures but not fluid and/or LH, you can still use that chart and replace the fluid or LH line with a custom tracking line.

You can also make a spreadsheet of your own, or utilize any apps which are comfortable and helpful for you. Just remember to not rely on an app to accurately predict fertility and/or your period date, and to do your own calculations to verify that ovulation has passed, since apps may not always calculate the same way you have been taught here.

If you end up working with an instructor in a specific method, please keep in mind that these Pearl and Thistle charts may not be suitable for the method! You should always defer to the proper protocols for observing, charting, and interpreting that match the method you are learning.

If you would like a digital copy of these charts, please submit a request to the author through pearlandthistle.com

Date																																													
Day of Cycle	1	2	3	4	5	6	7	8	9	10	11	12	13	14	15	16	17	18	19	20	21	22	23	24	25	26	27	28	29	30	31	32	33	34	35	36	37	38	39	40	41	42	43	44	45
	9	9	9	9	9	9	9	9	9	9	9	9	9	9	9	9	9	9	9	9	9	9	9	9	9	9	9	9	9	9	9	9	9	9	9	9	9	9	9	9	9	9	9	9	9
	8	8	8	8	8	8	8	8	8	8	8	8	8	8	8	8	8	8	8	8	8	8	8	8	8	8	8	8	8	8	8	8	8	8	8	8	8	8	8	8	8	8	8	8	8
	7	7	7	7	7	7	7	7	7	7	7	7	7	7	7	7	7	7	7	7	7	7	7	7	7	7	7	7	7	7	7	7	7	7	7	7	7	7	7	7	7	7	7	7	7
	6	6	6	6	6	6	6	6	6	6	6	6	6	6	6	6	6	6	6	6	6	6	6	6	6	6	6	6	6	6	6	6	6	6	6	6	6	6	6	6	6	6	6	6	6
Year	5	5	5	5	5	5	5	5	5	5	5	5	5	5	5	5	5	5	5	5	5	5	5	5	5	5	5	5	5	5	5	5	5	5	5	5	5	5	5	5	5	5	5	5	5
	4	4	4	4	4	4	4	4	4	4	4	4	4	4	4	4	4	4	4	4	4	4	4	4	4	4	4	4	4	4	4	4	4	4	4	4	4	4	4	4	4	4	4	4	4
________	3	3	3	3	3	3	3	3	3	3	3	3	3	3	3	3	3	3	3	3	3	3	3	3	3	3	3	3	3	3	3	3	3	3	3	3	3	3	3	3	3	3	3	3	3
	2	2	2	2	2	2	2	2	2	2	2	2	2	2	2	2	2	2	2	2	2	2	2	2	2	2	2	2	2	2	2	2	2	2	2	2	2	2	2	2	2	2	2	2	2
	1	1	1	1	1	1	1	1	1	1	1	1	1	1	1	1	1	1	1	1	1	1	1	1	1	1	1	1	1	1	1	1	1	1	1	1	1	1	1	1	1	1	1	1	1
	98	**98**	**98**	**98**	**98**	**98**	**98**	**98**	**98**	**98**	**98**	**98**	**98**	**98**	**98**	**98**	**98**	**98**	**98**	**98**	**98**	**98**	**98**	**98**	**98**	**98**	**98**	**98**	**98**	**98**	**98**	**98**	**98**	**98**	**98**	**98**	**98**	**98**	**98**	**98**	**98**	**98**	**98**	**98**	**98**
	9	9	9	9	9	9	9	9	9	9	9	9	9	9	9	9	9	9	9	9	9	9	9	9	9	9	9	9	9	9	9	9	9	9	9	9	9	9	9	9	9	9	9	9	9
	8	8	8	8	8	8	8	8	8	8	8	8	8	8	8	8	8	8	8	8	8	8	8	8	8	8	8	8	8	8	8	8	8	8	8	8	8	8	8	8	8	8	8	8	8
	7	7	7	7	7	7	7	7	7	7	7	7	7	7	7	7	7	7	7	7	7	7	7	7	7	7	7	7	7	7	7	7	7	7	7	7	7	7	7	7	7	7	7	7	7
	6	6	6	6	6	6	6	6	6	6	6	6	6	6	6	6	6	6	6	6	6	6	6	6	6	6	6	6	6	6	6	6	6	6	6	6	6	6	6	6	6	6	6	6	6
	5	5	5	5	5	5	5	5	5	5	5	5	5	5	5	5	5	5	5	5	5	5	5	5	5	5	5	5	5	5	5	5	5	5	5	5	5	5	5	5	5	5	5	5	5
	4	4	4	4	4	4	4	4	4	4	4	4	4	4	4	4	4	4	4	4	4	4	4	4	4	4	4	4	4	4	4	4	4	4	4	4	4	4	4	4	4	4	4	4	4
	3	3	3	3	3	3	3	3	3	3	3	3	3	3	3	3	3	3	3	3	3	3	3	3	3	3	3	3	3	3	3	3	3	3	3	3	3	3	3	3	3	3	3	3	3
Cycle #	2	2	2	2	2	2	2	2	2	2	2	2	2	2	2	2	2	2	2	2	2	2	2	2	2	2	2	2	2	2	2	2	2	2	2	2	2	2	2	2	2	2	2	2	2
	1	1	1	1	1	1	1	1	1	1	1	1	1	1	1	1	1	1	1	1	1	1	1	1	1	1	1	1	1	1	1	1	1	1	1	1	1	1	1	1	1	1	1	1	1
________	**97**	**97**	**97**	**97**	**97**	**97**	**97**	**97**	**97**	**97**	**97**	**97**	**97**	**97**	**97**	**97**	**97**	**97**	**97**	**97**	**97**	**97**	**97**	**97**	**97**	**97**	**97**	**97**	**97**	**97**	**97**	**97**	**97**	**97**	**97**	**97**	**97**	**97**	**97**	**97**	**97**	**97**	**97**	**97**	**97**
	9	9	9	9	9	9	9	9	9	9	9	9	9	9	9	9	9	9	9	9	9	9	9	9	9	9	9	9	9	9	9	9	9	9	9	9	9	9	9	9	9	9	9	9	9
	8	8	8	8	8	8	8	8	8	8	8	8	8	8	8	8	8	8	8	8	8	8	8	8	8	8	8	8	8	8	8	8	8	8	8	8	8	8	8	8	8	8	8	8	8
	7	7	7	7	7	7	7	7	7	7	7	7	7	7	7	7	7	7	7	7	7	7	7	7	7	7	7	7	7	7	7	7	7	7	7	7	7	7	7	7	7	7	7	7	7
	6	6	6	6	6	6	6	6	6	6	6	6	6	6	6	6	6	6	6	6	6	6	6	6	6	6	6	6	6	6	6	6	6	6	6	6	6	6	6	6	6	6	6	6	6
	5	5	5	5	5	5	5	5	5	5	5	5	5	5	5	5	5	5	5	5	5	5	5	5	5	5	5	5	5	5	5	5	5	5	5	5	5	5	5	5	5	5	5	5	5
	4	4	4	4	4	4	4	4	4	4	4	4	4	4	4	4	4	4	4	4	4	4	4	4	4	4	4	4	4	4	4	4	4	4	4	4	4	4	4	4	4	4	4	4	4
	3	3	3	3	3	3	3	3	3	3	3	3	3	3	3	3	3	3	3	3	3	3	3	3	3	3	3	3	3	3	3	3	3	3	3	3	3	3	3	3	3	3	3	3	3
	2	2	2	2	2	2	2	2	2	2	2	2	2	2	2	2	2	2	2	2	2	2	2	2	2	2	2	2	2	2	2	2	2	2	2	2	2	2	2	2	2	2	2	2	2
	1	1	1	1	1	1	1	1	1	1	1	1	1	1	1	1	1	1	1	1	1	1	1	1	1	1	1	1	1	1	1	1	1	1	1	1	1	1	1	1	1	1	1	1	1
	96	**96**	**96**	**96**	**96**	**96**	**96**	**96**	**96**	**96**	**96**	**96**	**96**	**96**	**96**	**96**	**96**	**96**	**96**	**96**	**96**	**96**	**96**	**96**	**96**	**96**	**96**	**96**	**96**	**96**	**96**	**96**	**96**	**96**	**96**	**96**	**96**	**96**	**96**	**96**	**96**	**96**	**96**	**96**	**96**

Day of Cycle	1	2	3	4	5	6	7	8	9	10	11	12	13	14	15	16	17	18	19	20	21	22	23	24	25	26	27	28	29	30	31	32	33	34	35	36	37	38	39	40	41	42	43	44	45
Period & Fluid																																													
Fluid Notations																																													
Period Pain?																																													
LH Tests (+/-)																																													
LH Notations																																													

KEY

Fluid Notations
L= Light Flow M= Moderate Flow H = Heavy Flow

Period & Fluid
P = flow of blood Dots = spotting O= dry, no fluid
⊖ = moist/sticky, pasty, creamy, slightly stretchy fluid
⊕= slippery/wet, clear, stretchy, slippery, watery fluid

Period Pain
0 = no pain
1 = a little uncomfortable
2 = medium amount of discomfort
3 = pain interferes with my day

LH Notations
X = invalid test

My Cycles This Past Year

Shortest Cycle ________ Longest Cycle ________

Shortest Period ________ Longest Period ________

Year: ______ Cycle #: ______

Date																																													

Day of Cycle	1	2	3	4	5	6	7	8	9	10	11	12	13	14	15	16	17	18	19	20	21	22	23	24	25	26	27	28	29	30	31	32	33	34	35	36	37	38	39	40	41	42	43	44	45
Period & Fluid																																													
Fluid Notations																																													
Period Pain?																																													
LH Tests (+/-)																																													
LH Notations																																													

KEY

<u>Fluid Notations</u>
L= Light Flow M= Moderate Flow H = Heavy Flow

<u>Period & Fluid</u>
P = flow of blood Dots = spotting O= dry, no fluid
⊖ = moist/sticky, pasty, creamy, slightly stretchy fluid
⊕= slippery/wet, dear, stretchy, slippery, watery fluid

<u>Period Pain</u>
0 = no pain
1 = a little uncomfortable
2 = medium amount of discomfort
3 = pain interferes with my day

<u>LH Notations</u>
X = invalid test

My Cycles This Past Year

Shortest Cycle ________ Longest Cycle ________
Shortest Period _____ Longest Period _____
Earliest LH Peak Day _______

Year: ______ Cycle #: ______

Date																																													

Day of Cycle	1	2	3	4	5	6	7	8	9	10	11	12	13	14	15	16	17	18	19	20	21	22	23	24	25	26	27	28	29	30	31	32	33	34	35	36	37	38	39	40	41	42	43	44	45
Period & Fluid																																													
Fluid Notations																																													
Period Pain?																																													
LH Tests (+/-)																																													
LH Notations																																													

KEY

<u>Fluid Notations</u>
L= Light Flow M= Moderate Flow H = Heavy Flow

<u>Period & Fluid</u>
P = flow of blood Dots = spotting O= dry, no fluid
⊖ = moist/sticky, pasty, creamy, slightly stretchy fluid
⊕= slippery/wet, dear, stretchy, slippery, watery fluid

<u>Period Pain</u>
0 = no pain
1 = a little uncomfortable
2 = medium amount of discomfort
3 = pain interferes with my day

<u>LH Notations</u>
X = invalid test

My Cycles This Past Year

Shortest Cycle ________ Longest Cycle ________
Shortest Period _____ Longest Period _____
Earliest LH Peak Day _______

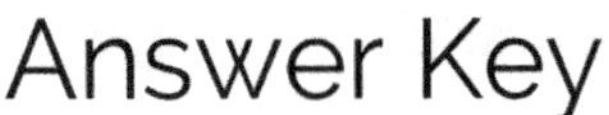

Answer Key

Charting Fluid, page 23

Tuesday

6:30 AM- moist, pasty white fluid
12 noon- moist, creamy white fluid
4:00 PM- wet, creamy white fluid
9:00 PM- wet, stretchy clear fluid
Today's category is: PEAK TYPE

Observation Category:
NON-PEAK
NON-PEAK
PEAK TYPE
PEAK TYPE

Moist, pasty, creamy, and white are all words in the Non-Peak category; but wet, stretchy, and clear are all Peak Type key words.

Wednesday

7:00 AM- wet, stretchy clear fluid
11:00 AM- wet, no fluid
3:30 PM- wet, no fluid
9:00 PM- wet, stretchy clear fluid
Today's category is: PEAK TYPE

Observation Category:
PEAK TYPE
PEAK TYPE
PEAK TYPE
PEAK TYPE

All of these observations were Peak Type, including those times when she didn't see anything ... because she still FELT wet.

Thursday

6:30 AM- moist, creamy white fluid
11:00 AM- moist, no fluid
3:30 PM- dry, no fluid
9:00 PM- dry, no fluid
Today's category is: NON-PEAK

Observation Category:
NON-PEAK
NON-PEAK
DRY
DRY

Moist, creamy, and white are all Non-Peak key words. Even though she trended towards Dry at the end of the day, it's still a Non-Peak day because of the earlier observations.

Adjusting Temperatures, page 26

Example 1

Base Time: 7:00 AM
Wake up time: 8:00 AM
Her thermometer read: 97.4°
She will chart: **97.2**

Example 2

Base Time: 7:00 AM
Wake up time: 8:30 AM
Her thermometer read: 97.8°
She will chart: **97.5**

Remember: if you wake up early, you need to ADD to that temp. If you wake up late, you need to SUBTRACT.

Example 3

Base Time: 7:00 AM
Wake up time: 6:30 AM
Her thermometer read: 97.7°
She will chart: **97.8**

Example 4

Base Time: 7:00 AM
Wake up time: 5:00 AM
Her thermometer read: 97.1°
She will chart: **97.5**

Terms to Know

Estrogen- one of the primary sex hormones that help develop and maintain female sex characteristics; within the context of a menstrual cycle, this hormone is responsible for cervical fluid production and endometrial development

Fallopian Tube- the tubes that extend on either side of the uterus toward the ovaries

Fertile Window- the time in a woman's menstrual cycle when a couple has the potential to conceive

Fertility Awareness Based Method (FABM)- a natural method of fertility management that includes tracking of biomarkers for ovulation. This could be considered a subset of NFP methods, although the two terms are often used interchangeably

Fibroids- muscular tumors that grow on the uterine wall

Fimbriae- fingerlike projections that extend from the Fallopian tube through which an egg would move from the ovary towards the uterus

Follicle- a fluid-filled sac within the ovary where an egg matures

Follicular Phase- the part of a menstrual cycle prior to ovulation during which an egg is maturing within a follicle

Follicle-Stimulating Hormone (FSH)- a hormone made by the pituitary gland that stimulates the growth of ovarian follicles

Gamete- a reproductive cell that contains half of the genetic information required to create a new person. The female gamete is the egg cell. The male gamete is the sperm cell.

Incarnation- a central Christian doctrine stating that the Son of God assumed human nature in the person of Jesus Christ

Language of the Body- a phrased used by Pope St. John Paul II to indicate the way our physical bodies express the nature and the reality of the person

LH Tests- urinary test strips that look for the presence of LH, which typically means that ovulation is likely about to happen

Luteal Phase- the part of the menstrual cycle after ovulation during which the *corpus luteum* secretes progesterone

Luteinized Unruptured Follicle (LUF)- when the dominant follicle fails to release its egg, but still transforms into a *corpus luteum*

Luteinizing Hormone (LH)- a pituitary hormone that stimulates ovulation

Terms to Know

Menopause- the natural cessation of menstrual cycles at the end of a woman's reproductive years

Menstrual Cup- flexible device that can be inserted into the vaginal canal to collect menstrual flow

Menstrual Cycle- the process of hormonal changes a woman's body undergoes in order to prepare for a possible pregnancy

Mystery- something that cannot be fully understood, because it is above our comprehension as a limited creature

Natural Family Planning (NFP)- a method of fertility management which does nothing before, during, or after an act of intercourse to render it sterile or incomplete

Oxytocin- often called the "love hormone," this neurotransmitter is involved in sexual arousal, parent-infant bonding during breastfeeding, and uterine contractions during labor

Ovulation- the release of a mature egg from the ovary

Peak Day- a term used in many NFP/FABM methods that helps identify ovulation. In this text, "Peak Day" is used to designate the last day of Peak Type fluid or the last day of a positive LH test to identify that ovulation has likely passed

Period- vaginal bleeding that occurs after successful ovulation in the absence of a pregnancy, also called menses or menstruation

Polycystic Ovary Syndrome (PCOS)- a medical condition related to high androgen production in women, often characterized by the presence of small fluid-filled sacs (cysts) in the ovaries

Polyps- overgrowths of uterine lining that can contribute to bleeding issues or infertility

Premenstrual Dysphoric Disorder (PMDD)- a very severe, often debilitating version of PMS

Premenstrual Syndrome (PMS)- signs and symptoms associated with the time leading up to a woman's period, which can range in intensity and duration. Severe PMS can interfere with daily activities and should be assessed with a doctor

Progesterone- a hormone secreted by the *corpus luteum* that prepares the endometrium for implantation during the latter part of the menstrual cycle and supports early stages of pregnancy

Restorative Reproductive Medicine- an approach that seeks to identify issues and correct underlying causes of reproductive and gynecological dysfunction

Sacrament- officially the seven Sacraments of the Catholic Church are those practices instituted by Christ that consist of outward signs through which divine grace is given. In a broader sense, this term can apply to any physical gesture or object—including the human body—that serves as a visible symbol of an invisible divine reality

Terms to Know

Urinary Metabolites- substances found within urine that are made when the body breaks down certain chemicals, including reproductive hormones

Uterus- also known as the womb, this female reproductive organ is located in the pelvis

Vagina- the internal muscular canal that extends from the vulva to the cervix

Vulva- the exterior part of female genitalia that includes the vaginal opening, urethral opening, labia, and clitoris

Yeast Infection- an overproduction of normally-occurring yeast that can cause vaginal itching, burning, and discharge

About Pearl & Thistle

Pearl & Thistle, LLC, was founded in 2018 by Christina Valenzuela, a certified NFP instructor with over a decade of coaching and parish ministry experience. Our mission is to provide an innovative approach to lifelong body literacy for Catholics, helping them share this information with their families, friends, and parishes.

At Pearl & Thistle, we believe that the Catholic Church is perfectly-poised to offer a synthesis between biology and theology, introducing girls and women to the *Language of the Body* in a way that helps them see their dignity from the very beginning stages of puberty and building upon that foundation as they grow.

If you would like to learn more about our work, please visit pearlandthistle.com

www.ingramcontent.com/pod-product-compliance
Lightning Source LLC
LaVergne TN
LVHW061252100826
845148LV00008B/1105

9798987213926